# AROMATHERAPY ANOINTING OILS
## SPIRITUAL BLESSINGS, CEREMONIES & AFFIRMATIONS

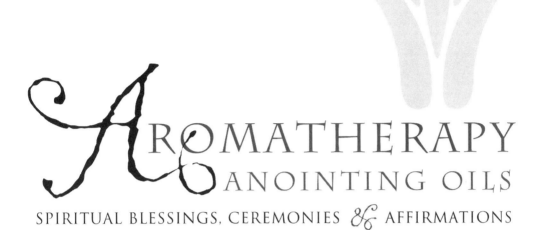

# AROMATHERAPY
## ANOINTING OILS
SPIRITUAL BLESSINGS, CEREMONIES & AFFIRMATIONS

JONI KEIM LOUGHRAN AND RUAH BULL

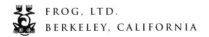

FROG, LTD.
BERKELEY, CALIFORNIA

# AROMATHERAPY ANOINTING OILS
## SPIRITUAL BLESSINGS, CEREMONIES & AFFIRMATIONS

Published by Frog, Ltd.
Frog, Ltd. Books are distributed by
North Atlantic Books
P O Box 12327
Berkeley, California 94712

Book cover and interior © 2001 Carolina de Bartolo.
Photos by Dennis K. Olsson.

North Atlantic Books are available through most bookstores. For further information, call 800-337-2665 or visit our website at www.northatlanticbooks.com.
Substantial discounts on bulk quantities are available to corporations, professional associations, and other organizations. For details and discount information, contact our special sales department.

Library of Congress Cataloging-in-Publication Data
Loughran, Joni.
    Aromatherapy anointing oils : spiritual blessings, ceremonies, and affirmations /
      by Joni Keim Loughran and Ruah Bull.
          p. cm.
    Includes index.
    ISBN 1-58394-045-6 (alk. paper)
      1. Essences and essential oils--Miscellanea. 2. Spiritual life--Miscellanea.
      3. Unction--Miscellanea. I. Bull, Ruah, 1951- II. Title.
BF1442.E77 L68 2001
291.4'46--dc21                              2001023815

1  2  3  4  5  6  7  8  9  /  04  03  02  01

# DEDICATIONS

## JONI

To my father who planted the first conceptual seeds of spirituality, knowing that one day they would flourish and I would find my way home.

## RUAH

To my mother, Kay, and father, Rich, who taught and showed me that spirituality is a part of every moment of every day.

# CONTENTS

# ACKNOWLEDGEMENTS

## JONI

My gratitude and appreciation to Dennis K. Olsson for his photography skills, his on-going support, and the countless hours of dialogue delving into the mystery of personal spirituality; Gail Atkins for her valuable editing skills; and Ruah Bull for enthusiastically rising to the occasion for this, our second book.

## RUAH

Thanks to all the women and men with whom I have sat in sacred circle during the past twenty years. I particularly want to thank Judy Zolezzi and Barbra Telynor—my co-teachers of The Winding Way, a spiritual studies program for women healers—for helping me remember ritual. Thanks to our good friend and colleague, The Reverend Margo Bearheart, for her assistance in Chapter 5. Finally, thanks to Joni for all the fun we have had in creating this book.

# FOREWORD

*A*s a pastor in what most would consider a fairly traditional, mainstream Protestant church, I find the use of anointing, aromatherapy, and other such practices relatively new, and even a bit strange, although they have been used in various forms for centuries. Though much of what I read in the pages of this book is unfamiliar, all of it is intriguing.

Some of the most prevalent voices I hear today, both within the church and without, are from people who are hungry to experience God. There is a growing interest in meditation, rituals, transforming prayers, and other spiritual practices. People don't just want to know about God or learn theological jargon; they want to personally know, be touched by, and experience God as directly as possible.

This book offers new ways to assist in this contemporary movement toward God and can enhance a journey of faith. As you read it, remember to keep separate the goal and the means to the goal. As we seek to know God more deeply, there are many practices and disciplines that can help us, but they will only be truly effective if we acknowledge them as aids, and not the primary experience. When used in this way, aromatherapy anointing and other techniques described in this book can provide support and inspiration for people of many spiritual and faith traditions to experience more profoundly the God of life. The authors present us with this opportunity as a gift, and invite us to partake.

THE REVEREND TIM KELLGREN
PETALUMA, CALIFORNIA, 2001

# INTRODUCTION

Spirituality is an integral and central part of human nature. *Aromatherapy Anointing Oils* is about experiencing, nurturing, and affirming spirituality through the ancient practice of anointing. Combined with the use of essential oils, the fragrant plant extracts used in aromatherapy, anointing offers a way to enrich and grace our spiritual path, inviting the sacred into our daily lives and helping us to shift our consciousness from the ordinary to the extraordinary.

Aromatherapy anointing is a spiritual blessing given to another, a group, or to ourselves. It is not the source or essence of the blessing—it is merely a tool to help visualize, amplify, and manifest the intention of it. Aromatherapy anointing can be used for everyday occasions such as beginning the day, or for special occasions such as a graduation or birthday.

In the last decade, there has been a fascinating shift in American religion and spirituality for which anointing is well-suited. Combined with the search for the mystical depths of spiritual nourishment is the desire to have our experiences be meaningful and vibrant, not only for ourselves, but also for our families and communities. Dogma may or may not be important, but there is an insistence that spirituality be alive and resonate with truth and personal meaning. Anointing addresses and embraces this very need and is a welcome addition to the ceremonies and rituals that express our faith and spiritual hopes and dreams.

We recognize that Americans, a diverse and multi-cultural group, experience their spiritual nature in unique and individual ways. Many who left the religion of their childhood during the social turbulence of the '60s and '70s later found themselves longing for, and returning to, their roots. Others have been drawn down paths of different cultures, especially those of Eastern, early European, and Native American traditions. Still others have embraced a combination of practices and beliefs from spiritual teachings gathered from around the world, as well as diverse disciplines such as transpersonal psychology and wholistic body therapies. There are also those who have remained faithfully engaged in their original religion.

In light of these different approaches, there are as many definitions of spirituality as there are spiritual practices. Yet within the amazing diversity that exists, we find common threads of agreement. In order to establish a foundational understanding of spirituality for the purpose of this book, we offer the following experiences as ones that we believe express the essence of human spirituality. These are often described by people on a spiritual path.

* Being aware of an intelligence, being, energy, force, or reality that is much vaster than our personal world. (Note: Throughout the book, we refer to this as Spirit, God, the Sacred, the Holy, and the Divine.)
* Being aware of the inter-relationship and connection of all life forms—an awareness that draws us to the practice of compassion, service, and love.
* Having a sense of meaning and purpose, coupled with the belief that there is goodness in the universe.
* Experiencing a joy and bliss from aligning our smaller selves with a greater plan, accessing—even for a moment—a Divine realm.
* Sensing the mystery of the Divine which is so beyond our human comprehension that we only experience glimpses of it, and may never be able to fully describe, analyze, or understand it.
* Longing to experience spirituality on a personal level.
* Believing that we *are* spiritual.

The intention of this book is to offer an avenue for experiencing spirituality in a personally meaningful way through the profound act of anointing combined with the remarkable qualities of essential oils. Both have a rich, historic past. Anointing has been used since ancient times for protection, recognition, devotion, and healing, by religious leaders and lay people alike. Essential oils, the perfect substances with which to anoint, have been used historically for this purpose. In addition, they have enticing fragrances that align with the ancient practice of using aroma to connect with the Divine, lifting our consciousness to a higher realm. As you explore anointing and essential oils together, we ask that you bring wisdom, self-awareness, and creativity to the process, using our information as a guide to enrich and evoke spiritual experiences in your daily life.

## CHAPTER ONE

# THE NATURE OF ANOINTING

*T*hroughout history, people have created ceremonies and customs within the context of their spiritual beliefs to celebrate, bless, and heal. One of the most common practices was, and still is, anointing, which simply means "to touch with oil." This ancient practice began when people trying to heal a wound swabbed it with oil. When healing took place, it was attributed to the particular deity revered by the people and was recognized as a bestowed favor. Oil became a symbol of the healing powers of the Divine, and anointing developed into an act of faith. In time, it represented the presence of the Divine in capacities other than healing, such as distinguishing someone chosen for a special purpose, or honoring someone for an accomplished task.

Anointing has evolved to represent a spiritual blessing—to dedicate and make sacred, to show Divine recognition, to request Divine favor, or to simply bestow goodness and grace. It is used not only for people, but also for animals, plants, objects, places, and events.

There are almost three hundred references to anointing in the Jewish and Christian Bibles. Kings, priests, and other prominent people were anointed to show their importance and commitment to God. The Psalms refer to the "oil of gladness." The prophet Isaiah speaks of the "oil of joy." Perhaps the most well-known story of anointing is that of Mary Magdalene, who anointed Jesus' head and feet with Spikenard to show her love and devotion to him. Anointing was also used for healing the sick, and many of Jesus' disciples were sent out to perform this task. The effects were believed to include not only physical healing, if God willed, but the restoration of spiritual well-being.

In the early years of the Christian church, anointing oils were blessed by a bishop, or someone in the role of spiritual leadership, and given to those in need. It became a means to offer Divine love, protection, and healing. Pope Innocent I said that once the oil was blessed, it was "lawful not for the priests only but for all Christians to use anointing in their own need or in the need of members of their household," bringing the practice of anointing into the realm of the lay person.

Other cultures and religions used anointing for similar purposes. Sometimes the person administering the anointing was a healer, or in a religious role, but often the anointing was performed by a friend or family member. In ancient Egypt, priests would oversee the anointing of mummies before burial, and the anointing of kings before they were crowned, for the purpose of Divine recognition. In India anointing the body with oil remains an integral part of the Hindu religion, as well as a component of Ayurveda, a five-thousand-year-old system of health care. Practiced by young and old in all walks of life, daily anointing is believed to help to maintain optimal health and to restore wellness for those who are ill.

## ANOINTING TODAY

The spiritual and religious tradition of anointing is as meaningful and important today as it has been for thousands of years. It remains an essential aspect of worship and is commonly used in religious contexts for baptism, confirmation, and ordination as well as for the dedication of churches and the blessing of altars and chalices.

Its uses, however, are evolving to meet the spiritual needs of contemporary people. Though rabbis, priests, monks, and shamans still use the ancient ritual as part of their religious duties, many are practicing anointing in new, creative, and non-traditional ways. For example, a minister and midwife offering comfort and healing to a woman who has experienced a miscarriage may rub the woman's belly with sage leaves, gently touching her body and blessing her with the oils released by the leaves.

Lay people create personal spiritual practices as a way to meaningfully integrate anointing into daily ritual and family ceremony. Someone hiking in the mountains picks up soil and touches her or his forehead to honor the sacredness of earth. A mother making dinner pours olive oil on the pasta with the intention of blessing the food, and a group of women anoints a pregnant friend at a baby shower. As more and more people discover and practice this ancient holy art, the uses and applications of anointing will continue to expand.

Shared in the following experiences are unique perspectives and understandings of anointing. One massage therapist, before giving a massage, enters into a spiritual state of mind as a form of anointing. A musician who performs in hospitals perceives her music as a type of anointing. A teacher notices that anointing both the student and a specially chosen object helps to manifest personal goals. The common thread running through these personal accounts is the awareness that anointing is not an end in itself, but rather a means to shift consciousness and focus in order to experience a closer relationship with the Divine.

Traditionally, anointing was performed by one person to another, such as a healer anointing a sick child, or a shaman anointing a chief. However, today, self-anointing is an honored practice in which the giver and receiver of the blessing are one.

## JUDY ZOLEZZI

Judy is a spiritual director and a skilled massage therapist. She honors all spiritual paths and believes in the "golden thread" of mercy, love, compassion, healing, forgiveness, and peace that weaves through them all. Her personal path is one that embraces the wisdom and teachings of Christ and Buddha—an East-meets-West way of approaching life each day.

As a massage practitioner, before each session begins, Judy blesses the oil, linens, table, and room. Then she anoints the entire body of her client with oil, lights a candle, and offers a prayer. "For me, anointing is about a whole way of being. It's about how I am with the person—blessing, honoring, revering, and respecting the sacredness of the body. All of this is conveyed through the simple act of touch. I hold a certain sacred quality of presence so that after the session, the client is more conscious of having been blessed." In her experience of reverence, both she and her client are anointed.

Judy believes that anointing goes beyond the use of a particular oil. "We can anoint, bless, and honor someone with our eyes, our voice, our hands, and our entire self." She reminds us about the importance of intention—the knowing and clarity of purpose—behind an anointing, and she expands our understanding of this spiritual practice to encompass our whole being. She invites us to imagine ourselves as a sacred oil that can heal, bless, and awaken to Spirit all that we touch.

## BARBRA TELYNOR

Barbra Telynor is a former Congregational minister who now works as a harpist and "midwife of the soul" for several local hospitals. She uses music and ceremony to assist people in the process of healing, and of dying. Barbra calls herself a "contemporary ritualist," and she helps people design personal ceremonies for which she will officiate, such as a career change or graduation.

Barbra perceives anointing as "a blessing that recognizes the sacred wholeness of the person—whether it is with music, water, or oil." She uses her music to anoint the environment, creating a sacred space and time. She finds music particularly helpful in changing the ambience in a hospital room. During her specially designed ceremonies she may also use different types of water for anointing. River water is chosen when someone needs help to progress or to "flow along" on his/her life journey, and ocean water helps to deepen the understanding of a particular situation. She uses essential oil of Lavender to bring clarity and balance for someone facing major life changes, such as divorce.

Barbra believes that ritual, and the anointing that is a part of it, is "preparation for the work at hand. It creates the space, then the work follows." She smiles. For Barbra, anointing provides support for what is to come—whether it is music filling the room of a dying person, a spray of water landing upon the about-to-be-wed couple's heads at a marriage, or a drop of oil placed on the hands of a sculptor.

LAURA BINAH FELDMAN

Laura Binah is a ceremonialist, storyteller, and teacher who refers to herself as a Pagan Jew. Her beliefs recognize the presence of the Divine everywhere, and she practices a nature-based Judaism that honors the pagan roots of the Jewish religion. She explains that Judaism and Paganism share a belief that the ordinary and the sacred are not mutually exclusive—that ritual, awareness, intention, and prayer transform even the most mundane events and routines into holiness, allowing us to live richer, more harmonious lives.

Laura Binah says that anointing with oil is a traditional Jewish practice. Historically, the high priest was anointed for temple service in Jerusalem. However, she uses anointing to turn simple, daily acts into sacred occasions. For example, in Judaism, before eating bread, one washes their hands by using a cup of water, pouring it three times over each hand, and then raising their hands while reciting a blessing. In her own home, Laura Binah adds essential oil to the water for hand washing, selecting an aroma appropriate for the season or occasion. Anointing is particularly compatible with the traditional Jewish teaching that states, "You should say one hundred blessings a day." Blessings can include gesture and words, as well as touch.

Laura Binah performs both traditional and non-traditional anointing for her community in a variety of ways. She is a member of her temple's Holy Society, whose sacred task is preparing the dead for burial. Part of the traditional ritual preparation includes ceremonial washing and anointing with soil from the land of Israel just before the coffin is closed. Non-traditionally, she uses essential oils combined for the occasion to anoint couples for wedding blessings and for women participating in new moon ceremonies.

By anointing with both simple substances such as water and ethereal substances such as essential oils, Laura feels there is a blessed joining of the Earth and the heavens.

## PHYLLIS WILLIAMS

Phyllis Williams is a Reiki practitioner, and she teaches classes in candle rituals. She incorporates anointing with essential oils in her private Reiki sessions, her classes, and in her personal life.

Phyllis notices that changes in people's lives as well as seasonal shifts are reflected in the essential oils that her clients and students choose. In fall and winter, people are drawn to the oils that support "going inward" such as Sandalwood or Frankincense. In spring and summer, people choose energizing oils that support creative, outward expression such as Rosemary or Peppermint.

For a Reiki session, Phyllis rubs the client's chosen oil on her hands. She then moves her hands lightly over their head and gently touches the Third Eye, a place between the eyebrows. Later in the session, with the oil still on her hands, she kneads the feet, with particular attention to the area on the big toe that relates to the pituitary gland associated with the Third Eye. She believes that the pituitary gland, also known as the master gland, is the "place where everything starts," and so she begins and ends her sessions with an anointing touch to stimulate and support it.

In Phyllis' candle ritual classes, students anoint both themselves and the candle with a chosen essential oil. She believes that this dual anointing helps the person become more fully aware of their intention so that personal power and focus can manifest the desired effect. Phyllis describes what happens in this process. "We take responsibility for our own growth. We take the first step with intention, we awaken the God energy within, and then God can help."

Phyllis also uses essential oils for personal anointing in her daily life, placing a few drops of Rose oil into her bath to release all negativity and bring unconditional love into her life. She uses oils both to anoint her body and to diffuse in a room to create a sacred and healing environment.

JAN BODDIE AND MARYSTELLA CHURCH

Jan Boddie, Ph.D., psychotherapist, and Marystella Church, intuitive energy healer, work together to create sacred ceremonies for healing and celebrating the personal and collective relationship with Spirit. They have both studied with Malidoma and Sobonfu Somé of West Africa. In the Dagara tradition of the Somés' homeland, the five elements of Fire, Water, Earth, Nature, and Mineral are a part of every ritual. Fire represents our spontaneity and passion, and connects us with our ancestors. Water is cleansing and represents the flow of movement that finds its way around obstacles. Earth represents home, abundance, and visibility. Nature is the symbol of authenticity and transition, often called upon to assist in removing the mask we wear when we are resistant to change. Minerals represent our memories and connect us to ancient wisdom. Marystella explains that the element Air, which in Western tradition symbolizes Spirit, "is not included by the Dagara tribe because they believe Spirit is everywhere, all the time." Jan and Marystella use the tradition of anointing to help us remember this presence of Spirit.

Jan, who loves etymology or word derivation, discovered that "anointing" not only means to touch with oil, but also to smear, to consecrate, or to make sacred in ceremony. "Anointing plays a role in many of our rites and rituals. It's a powerful, symbolic action because symbols are the language of our psyche. Anointing is a wake-up call, facilitating a conscious connection with the parts of ourselves that have been lost or forgotten."

Together, Jan and Marystella share how anointing is used in their work. "Sometimes we dip a feather in sea water, then touch each person's forehead. Sea salt is a symbol of purification in many cultures, and the anointing action, combined with the physical sensation of softness and wetness, awakens intention—the yearning to connect with Spirit. Sometimes we anoint by washing each person's feet, often with a few drops of Lavender oil in the water to complement the symbolic action of cleansing the past and clearing the present path. One of our favorite ways to anoint is to use mud by making designs on the face, arms, and hands. Mud combines the power of earth, a symbol of home as the sacred center within each individual, with the power of water."

Ritual creates a sacred space for people to both give and receive the blessings of anointing, a powerful tool for connecting and remembering our relationship with Self, Others, Spirit, and Earth. Jan writes in her book, *Circle Left to Enter Rite,* "Private ritual, which helps us to honor the Self and heal the inner Spirit, provides the sustenance for connecting authentically with the greater collective. Community ritual helps us to heal the split between me and you, us and them, providing the sustenance for connecting authentically with the Self."

## MARGO BEARHEART

The Reverend Margo Bearheart is a spiritual teacher, energy healer, and a sacred wisdom-way teacher—a person initiated in the sacred healing and spiritual teachings of cross-cultural shamanism. She has studied with several medicine teachers and spent seven years as an apprentice to a medicine elder. She is the founder and director of the Transformational and Healing Arts Center in Santa Rosa, California.

Margo uses anointing in all of her work—classes, healing sessions, and ceremonies—but primarily for blessings and dedications. Margo says that blessings open the way for Spirit to enter. This allows the object of the blessing—person, place, or thing—to be touched by and filled with Spirit. Dedication is the process of setting a specific intention. For example, when students graduate from her programs, each one declares their intention, stating their purpose and the path to which they are dedicating themselves.

Margo uses anointing as a part of the opening and closing of a blessing, and to acknowledge and confirm a dedication. She does this by smudging (cleansing and purifying with smoke) the room with the herb of sage, and then sprinkling the area and the participants with a cedar branch that has been dipped in water infused with essential oils—usually Sandalwood, Cedarwood, Rose, or Sage.

She also incorporates anointing at the end of a healing session in which she has worked on the energy centers (chakras). She places an appropriate essential oil into a bowl of water and then anoints the energy center herself, or has the client anoint the center while they talk about their healing intention out loud. She believes that the combination of water, essential oil, touch, and speech creates a powerful matrix for healing.

## OUR DEFINITION OF ANOINTING

As we see from the above descriptions, anointing is used in a spiritual context for many purposes, and in many settings and ways. Its traditional and historical use for blessing and healing is still practiced, yet its applications have changed and flourished to nourish today's spiritual longings and needs.

The simple yet profound practice of anointing or "touching with oil" lends itself to creativity, imagination, and intention. We teach that anointing is a *spiritual practice*—uncomplicated, easy, and natural. It captures and embraces a spiritual focus, much the same as we do in prayer or meditation. It is done *with a special substance, in a sacred space and time, in a certain way, for a specific purpose.* Each act of anointing, as a symbolic action infused with intention, provides an opportunity to give and receive blessings, as well as to visualize and manifest goals for personal and spiritual growth.

CHAPTER TWO
# ESSENTIAL OILS FOR ANOINTING

*A*s mentioned at the end of Chapter 1, anointing is a spiritual practice that uses *a special substance, in a sacred space and time, in a certain way, for a specific purpose.* In this chapter, we explore the premier "special substance" for anointing—essential oils. Though other substances can be used, there is nothing more perfect than these precious plant extracts. They have been used historically for anointing. Their exquisite fragrances lift and focus our consciousness. In addition, they are the cornerstone of aromatherapy, a natural, wholistic health care modality that promotes wellness on physical, psychological, and subtle energy levels. (Subtle energy anatomy, the energy centers, and the subtle bodies are described in Chapter 4.)

## THE NATURE OF ESSENTIAL OILS

Essential oils are highly concentrated plant extracts. They exist in a variety of fragrances (very sweet to highly pungent), a variety of colors (crystal clear to dark amber), and a variety of viscosities (thin and watery to thick and syrupy). Many of them are volatile, evaporating into the air if left in an open container. This volatility is why essential oils have often been called ethereal oils, which means "pertaining to the heavens"—a term that is particularly appropriate for anointing.

Various plant parts such as the flowers, leaves, roots, seeds, wood, and rinds produce essential oils. Which part or parts are used depends on the plant. For example, essential oil of Rose is from the flowers, Orange is from the rinds, and Vetiver is from the roots. To extract the essential oil from a particular plant, the method chosen must best preserve the oil's valuable therapeutic properties at the right stage of plant development. Steam distillation is used for most plants, though cold-expression extraction is used for citrus rinds. Other methods include the use of solvents and carbon dioxide.

Essential oils are wholistic in their actions—they influence all realms of human nature. Let us take for example Lavender: on a physical level it relieves the pain of a burn, on a psychological level it relaxes and stabilizes, and on a subtle energy level it balances all the energy centers and promotes spiritual growth. Essential oils are well-suited for self-care but have also been internationally embraced by professionals in the medical, chiropractic, alternative health, physical therapy, psychology, cosmetology, and religious communities.

Because essential oils are so highly concentrated, they are diluted before use, whether it is for a physical, psychological, or subtle energy purpose. Undiluted oils can be irritating to the skin. When working with essential oils on a physical level or for a psychological response, the standard recommended dilution is two percent. In the case of essential oils, more is not necessarily better. When working with essential oils for anointing, we recommend using them in a one percent or less dilution, to focus the impact on the subtle energy level rather than on the physical or psychological realms.

Essential oils are therapeutically effective only if they are pure, unadulterated, and extracted from plants that have been properly grown, harvested, and distilled. Most essential oils are complex, and their unique restorative properties cannot be synthetically duplicated in a laboratory.

Be aware that when you are using essential oils, there are safety guidelines to follow. We suggest obtaining one of the books listed in Resources to use as a reference. See Appendix I for general safety recommendations.

## HOW ESSENTIAL OILS AFFECT US

When using essential oils for anointing, we draw upon their fragrance and their subtle energy (or energetic/vibrational) qualities. Our sense of smell as well as our energy field and centers respond to these properties.

Fragrance has long been used by many cultures in a sacred context as an offering to the heavens, as a connection with the Divine, and to assist with healing, prayer, and meditation. This association of the spiritual realm with fragrance is deeply rooted in tradition and is still practiced today. Incense is commonly burned in Christian churches and Buddhist shrines. Native Americans use fragrant herbs placed on hot rocks in their sweat lodges to facilitate a spiritual connection, and Tibetans burn bundles of juniper to accompany their prayers.

When scent is inhaled through the nose, certain odor molecules enter the lungs and others travel to the brain. Via the lungs, the odor molecules enter the blood stream and circulate through the body. Those traveling to the brain are perceived by our sense of smell and have a profound effect, producing and evoking emotional and physical responses as well as memories. When specific fragrances are used with a spiritual intent, the connection and experience are stored in our brain and remembered. When the fragrance is smelled again, it evokes a spiritual response. The more a fragrance is used, the stronger the connection becomes.

The subtle energy nature of essential oils primarily affects our subtle anatomy—the electromagnetic field and energy centers—though physical and psychological states are also affected due to the wholistic nature of both human beings and essential oils. The subtle qualities of the oils can assist us in every aspect of our lives, from feeling secure in the world to following our spiritual path, helping us achieve a state of balance and sense of well-being. They are especially useful for meditation, affirmations, and visualizations.

The subtle energy qualities of essential oils are utilized by the field of vibrational medicine, which is based on the awareness that all matter is energy. Everything has an electromagnetic field that vibrates in a particular way. Each life form has its own healthy vibrational signature, which changes in the presence of illness or imbalance. Researcher Dr. Valerie Hunt has studied and described the electromagnetic field of the human body, which she calls the biofield. In her book, *The Infinite Mind,* there are illustrations of this field in both its healthy (balanced) and unhealthy (unbalanced) states. Barbara Brennan's book, *Hands of Light*, also has excellent illustrations. This biofield can be referred to as the *subtle bodies* or *energy field*, terms that are more commonly used.

Essential oils are used to affect the subtle anatomy by gently coaxing erratic cellular vibration back to its original healthy pattern via *persuasive resonance*. Many essential oils vibrate in harmony with the energy centers and therefore can be used to assist in returning the centers to balance.

Those who work with essential oils and are particularly attuned to them, perceive them as unique and precious substances. Malte Hozzel, a naturalist and purveyor of essential oils, describes them as "carriers of light." Gabriel Mojay, author of *Aromatherapy for Healing the Spirit*, depicts them as messengers of energy and consciousness. Valerie Ann Worwood, author of *Fragrant Heavens*, believes that essential oils help us to contact "the wisdom of nature, the power of light, the energy of the universe, and the love in our hearts."

Through historic and traditional use, the impact of their fragrance, their role in vibrational medicine, and personal experience, we see how essential oils are ultimately perfect for amplifying the intention of sacred anointing.

## THE ESSENTIAL OILS: A TO Z
The essential oils listed below are profiled in six categories to give you a broad range of understanding and application when using essential oils for subtle energy purposes, and most specifically for anointing.

SPIRITUAL TEACHINGS refers to the lessons and stages of the spiritual path and human journey as conveyed by the oil.

OCCASIONS FOR USE describes psychological/spiritual states that would benefit from the oil.

ENERGY CENTERS refers to the seven major energy vortices that are aligned along our spine.

PHYSICAL SITES notes the parts of the body associated with psychological states that would be appropriate for anointing.

BLESSINGS are prayerful calls to Spirit to fulfill our personal intention.

AFFIRMATIONS are positive statements that name your intention to support and strengthen the efficacy of the self.

If there are terms in the descriptions that are unfamiliar to you, please review the Glossary, Appendix II.

As you are learning this information, please keep in your mind and heart that it has been filtered through our, the authors', consciousness. This means that the teachings perceived are ones we were *able* to perceive. You may have a different perception and experience. A part of the extraordinary power of these oils is their ability to tailor their messages to each individual, approaching us with palpable wisdom and respect. Also, you will notice that some of the oils have similar teachings. This list will give you the opportunity to find the oil whose fragrance and idiosyncrasies you prefer.

Included in each essential oil profile is the Latin or botanical name of the plant from which the essential oil is extracted, the part of the plant that is used, and the common geographical location where the plant is grown.

---

*Note: Many of the essential oils are familiar, and easy to find in natural food stores. Others are rare and uncommon, but are available by mail order. See Resources.*

# ANGELICA *(Angelica archangelica)* ROOT
HUNGARY

## SPIRITUAL TEACHINGS

Angelica teaches us that we are not alone. There are celestial beings who watch over and protect us. Many religious traditions, including Judeo-Christian, Muslim, and Buddhist, teach about angels. They are described as "messengers of God" or "beings of light" who are always present. Some angels are guardians who speak to us, surround us, and enfold us in their wings during times of trouble. Others bring messages and blessings from Spirit—the highest source of wisdom.

Angelica assists in bringing us into conscious relationship with the angelic realm so we can receive its teachings, benefit from its wisdom, and draw sustenance and courage from knowing that the angels protect and guide us. This oil also brings us into alliance with our higher self so we are better able to accept the angels' gifts of kindness and compassion and to represent them in the world.

## OCCASIONS FOR USE

To bring light and wisdom into our life.

To experience the presence of angels.

To become a source of illumination and love in the lives of others.

During meditation to provide protection from outside influences, and to connect with angelic guidance.

## ENERGY CENTERS

Seventh: Connects us with angelic guidance. Encourages the presence of angels. Strengthens the spirit. Aligns us with our higher self. Balances and protects us during meditative states.

First: Grounds.

PHYSICAL SITES
Base of skull, top of head.

BLESSINGS
May the angels bless me, hold me, and keep me safe.
May I be filled with angelic light so that I may be a source of light for others.
May I know and act from my higher self.

AFFIRMATIONS
I am open to receiving angelic guidance.
I am a source of love and light.

## ANISE *(Pimpinella anisum)* PLANT
### TURKEY / SPAIN

SPIRITUAL TEACHINGS
In some esoteric traditions there is a metaphysical teaching that recognizes thoughts as actual objects—they have form, energy, and enormous impact. Called "thoughtforms," they represent our perceptions and beliefs about reality, determine how we experience life, and draw experiences to us that confirm our belief system. For example, if we believe that all people are unkind, then we are going to notice unkind people and their actions. We may not notice or give credence to other ways in which people act. We will also draw unkind people to us, unconsciously, to confirm our beliefs.

Part of the challenge on the spiritual path is to identify and release stereotypical, judgmental, or preconceived ideas about the world around us, other people, and ourselves. This frees the mind to create new beliefs and expectations that are more positive. Anise assists in clearing out old, outmoded thoughtforms that are not beneficial. By releasing them, a more enlightened, compassionate, loving, and true self can emerge.

## OCCASIONS FOR USE

During times of mental confusion, particularly when plagued by obsessive, negative, or limiting thoughts.

To release old spiritual beliefs.

To assist us in changing any aspect of our life that is hindering our personal and spiritual growth.

## ENERGY CENTERS

General: Clears and cleanses the energy field so that energy can move easily through the various subtle bodies, working with the mental level to increase mental clarity.

Seventh and Sixth: Clears away old thoughtforms so spiritual information can be received.

## PHYSICAL SITES

Top of head, temples, solar plexus.

## BLESSINGS

May my life be connected to the Divine source.

May my mind be filled with the light, love, and truth of Spirit.

May my mind be clear and positive.

## AFFIRMATIONS

I am free of any thoughts, ideas, or beliefs that no longer serve me.

My mind is healed and balanced.

## AZALEA *(Azalea)* BLOSSOMS

FRANCE

## SPIRITUAL TEACHINGS

Humans experience a wide range of emotions such as fear, love, sadness, joy, anger, and compassion. Many emotions are helpful and necessary, providing us with important information about our experiences as well as our perception of experiences. However, our emotions can also prevent us from thinking and perceiving clearly, and from living in the present moment. For example, if we react with fear in a situation that reminds us (consciously or unconsciously) of a previous frightening experience, these old feelings keep us from knowing what is actually happening.

Azalea helps us develop emotional wisdom in relationship to spiritual truth, enabling us to respond as authentically as possible to the here and now. Emotions that bind us to the past or propel us into the future can be gently and effectively released by Azalea. When these emotions are released, we are able to truly connect with ourselves and others, and to receive and understand the spiritual teachings being presented to us.

## OCCASIONS FOR USE
During times of turbulent emotions to stay connected to spiritual guidance.
When our emotions overtake us in ways that harm ourselves or others.
During times of emotional healing and growth.

## ENERGY CENTERS
General: Helps to integrate masculine and feminine energies.
Seventh: Releases emotions lodged in the subtle bodies that interfere with receiving
    spiritual guidance and prevent us from knowing our spiritual path.

## PHYSICAL SITES
Heart, full length of back, left and right side of body.

## BLESSINGS
May my emotions be true teachers.
May I be receptive to spiritual guidance during this emotional time.
May all outmoded emotions be released so that I may experience my true feelings in
    each moment.

AFFIRMATIONS
I release all stagnated emotions.
I observe and learn from my emotions.
My emotions lead me to Spirit.

## BAY LAUREL *(Laurus nobilis)* LEAVES
### CROATIA

### SPIRITUAL TEACHINGS
There is a spiritual/metaphysical concept that states, "Energy follows thought." This indicates that our thoughts create reality, having an enormous impact on our lives. For example, if you think that you are not intelligent, you may, consciously or unconsciously, create difficulties for yourself in learning environments. When you do learn something, you may discount that achievement because it does not match your perception of yourself. In other words, on a subtle level, we are what we think we are. It follows, then, that when we change our thoughts, we change our reality and experiences. Bay Laurel strengthens our intuition, helps to release old, outmoded thoughts about ourselves, and energetically prepares us so that we can receive and integrate new beliefs into our minds and hearts.

### OCCASIONS FOR USE
To help identify and/or release thought patterns about ourselves that harm or limit.
To support affirmations.
To help identify the thought behind a feeling.
To become more intuitive.

### ENERGY CENTERS
Sixth: Promotes psychic awareness and intuition. Provides psychic protection. Opens
us to new thoughts and perspectives. Releases mental blocks and outmoded beliefs.

PHYSICAL SITES

Temples, solar plexus, joints.

BLESSINGS

May I release all negative thoughts.

May my mind be open to positive change.

May my thoughts energize, heal, and transform me.

AFFIRMATIONS

I release all negative thoughts.

I choose the thoughts that support my unfolding spiritual path.

I am intuitive.


BENZOIN *(Styrax benzoe)* RESIN

INDONESIA

SPIRITUAL TEACHINGS

Many traditions acknowledge that one of the highest goals on the spiritual path is compassionate wisdom. In order to develop the wise heart, we need to be aware of our emotional wounds, past and present, and begin the process of healing and releasing them. Benzoin provides comfort, love, and support during this process. It teaches us to accept all of our emotions, allowing all thoughts and feelings to be witnessed, and then gently released. It teaches us to have compassion for ourselves and our past, helping us to grow slowly and deeply in wisdom.

OCCASIONS FOR USE

To help us release painful emotions.

When we are impatient about our progress on our spiritual path.

To give us courage in facing the task of self-improvement.

ENERGY CENTERS

General: Dispels anger and negativity.

Sixth: Provides psychic protection. Steadies and focuses the mind for meditation or prayer. Allows buried thoughts and feelings to come safely to consciousness to be examined and processed. Helps us to become aware of our true thoughts and feelings.

Fourth: Comforts and soothes. Encourages self-compassion.

First: Grounds and comforts, especially during psychological "releasing" experiences.

PHYSICAL SITES

Feet, hips, joints.

BLESSINGS

May I feel and know my true feelings.

May all stagnated energy that does not benefit me be released.

May my heart be filled with compassion.

May my mind be blessed with wisdom.

AFFIRMATIONS

I practice compassion for myself.

I am growing and healing.

I embrace and embody the wise heart.

# BERGAMOT *(Citrus bergamia)* RIND

IVORY COAST

SPIRITUAL TEACHINGS

Bergamot supports and lightens the grieving heart. It allows our feelings to heal in their own time and rhythm. It provides comfort while encouraging fortitude and courage, helping us to move through the numbness and the suffering. When we emerge from this experience, Bergamot offers a sense of completion, encouraging us to embrace all of life's experiences with joy in our heart.

Bergamot also helps us to accept our physical body. In Western culture today, many people, particularly women, are overly critical of the size and shape of their bodies. Unrealistic and even dangerous ideals are held out as a goal. Bergamot helps us to embrace our imperfections and delight in our unique beauty—our perfectly imperfect bodies—to understand that the body is the physical home for our spirit.

OCCASIONS FOR USE
To help us experience and deal with grief.
When we feel overwhelmed with grief or sadness.
To help recover from negative feelings about one's body.
To appreciate the body as the temple and expression of the Divine.

ENERGY CENTERS
General: Brings in positive energy.
Fourth: Supports self-love. Opens the Heart center and allows love to radiate.
    Eases grief.
First: Supports love for one's physical body.

PHYSICAL SITES
Heart, upper back, knee.

BLESSINGS
I offer this unbearable feeling of grief to Spirit.
Help me to bear this grief.
May I care for my body from a place of deep love.

AFFIRMATIONS
I honor my grief.
I embrace all of life's experiences with joy.

I accept my body in its uniquely perfect imperfections.
My body is an expression of the Divine.

## BLACK PEPPER *(Piper nigrum)* FRUIT
### SRI LANKA

### SPIRITUAL TEACHINGS

As we grow spiritually, we may experience unresolved past or present anger and/or frustration. All strong emotions have their purpose. Anger is intended to notify us and protect us when we are being physically or psychologically assaulted. It gives us important information that something is wrong, that we may be harmed, and that we need to react. Once having served its purpose, anger should be acknowledged, respected, and then released. If not, it creates physical stiffness, emotional disconnection, mental rigidity, and spiritual aridity.

Black Pepper helps us deal with anger and gives us the courage to do so. It supports us when we are feeling angry, helps us react appropriately, and then allows us to let it go. In the letting go, we become more fully open to Spirit.

### OCCASIONS FOR USE

During times of anger or frustration.
To help us release anger.
To give us courage in facing our unresolved anger.

### ENERGY CENTERS

General: Dissolves energy blockages caused by anger and frustration.
Third: Increases courage.

### PHYSICAL SITES

Solar plexus, heart, temples, buttocks, joints.

BLESSINGS

May I comfortably and honestly release old anger and frustration.

May I be blessed and protected as I release my anger and frustration.

May I use my anger to grow and heal.

AFFIRMATIONS

I am courageous in facing my unresolved anger or frustration.

I release the anger that no longer serves me.

I acknowledge my anger as a gift to teach me and help me grow.


# CAJEPUT *(Melaleuca cajuputii)* LEAVES
### INDONESIA

SPIRITUAL TEACHINGS

Jesus taught his followers to be like little children—to trust God in the same way that a loved child trusts its parents. This creates an innocence that is encouraged by Spirit and filled with devotion. It helps us to submit to the trials as well as the delights of the spiritual path. When we place our trust in Spirit, we believe all that happens is for the unfolding of our higher selves. Cajeput helps to evoke this child-like innocence, reminding us that we are loved and safe in the world.

OCCASIONS FOR USE

When feeling scared.

To develop trust and faith.

During times of change.

ENERGY CENTERS

General: Connects us with child-like devotion to trust in the universe.

Seventh: Supports and encourages devotion to Spirit.

Third: Helps us to trust ourselves.
First: Promotes a sense of security and trust in the world.

PHYSICAL SITES
Base of skull, shoulders, solar plexus.

BLESSINGS
Bless the child within me.
May I be filled with trust and devotion.
May I have faith and trust during times of change.
May I feel the presence of Divine love and assistance.

AFFIRMATIONS
I am safe.
I have all that I need.
I know that I am loved.


CALAMUS *(Acorus calamus)* PLANT

CANADA

SPIRITUAL TEACHINGS
Calamus assists in the emergence of contemporary spirituality—the teaching, sharing, and integration of many paths and traditions. It is useful for those who are called upon to share their spiritual experiences or insights with others, whether personally or professionally. It helps us to speak about our spirituality in ways that are respectful of others' beliefs and experiences. In this way we can touch and even heal others with our words. It also enables us to listen deeply to others. The wise use of words, the art of listening, and the insight of silence are invaluable for respecting today's wide variety of spiritual experiences.

## OCCASIONS FOR USE

To communicate our spiritual understanding in a clear and respectful way.

To support spiritual growth and sharing, in a group or class.

To release feelings of being offended or hurt by another's spiritual beliefs or words.

## ENERGY CENTERS

General: Good for any kind of spiritual/intuitive work. Promotes spiritual understanding and communication.

Seventh: Initiates the reception of spiritual information, enabling us to know our highest truth.

Sixth: Helps us to clearly understand our spiritual experiences.

Fifth: Helps us to clearly communicate our spiritual experiences.

## PHYSICAL SITES

Temples, throat, feet.

## BLESSINGS

May I hear and speak the highest truth.

May I learn when to speak, when to listen, and when to enter silence.

## AFFIRMATIONS

I speak the truth, respecting myself and others.

I honor my spiritual path and the paths of others.

I am open to understanding other ideas and philosophies.

## CEDARWOOD *(Cedrus atlantica)* WOOD

MOROCCO

## SPIRITUAL TEACHINGS

One of the most powerful essential oils for subtle energy work, Cedarwood is grounding, clears away negativity, and brings in positive energy. It promotes clarity of mind and invokes the presence and teachings of the Divine. Whatever holy teaching is needed is accessed by this direct link to the Divine—a link that supercedes all other guidance.

## OCCASIONS FOR USE

When feeling ungrounded.

When feeling negativity from other people or ourselves.

During times of spiritual confusion—not knowing what we believe.

For meditation to help connect us with Spirit.

## ENERGY CENTERS

General: Clears and cleanses a room. Brings in positive energy.

Seventh: Restores a sense of spiritual certainty. Strengthens the connection with the Divine.

Sixth: Clears and steadies the mind. Promotes a calm meditative state.

Third: Strengthens confidence and will.

First: Connects us with earthly forces. Grounds.

## PHYSICAL SITES

Temples, solar plexus, feet.

## BLESSINGS

May I be filled with Divine love, breath, and wisdom.

May this space be cleared of all negativity.

May I have a clear mind to receive Divine teachings.

## AFFIRMATIONS

I am grounded.

I have all the strength and confidence that I need.

My mind is clear to receive and recognize spiritual truths.

## CHAMOMILE, GERMAN *(Chamomilla matricaria)* FLOWERING PLANT
NEPAL

### SPIRITUAL TEACHINGS

A great spiritual presence is that of the visionary, defined by anthropologist Angeles Arrien as the one who speaks the truth without blame or judgement. We have a sacred task to discover truth in any given moment. German Chamomile helps us to identify what is true, and also to find a way to speak it with grace, accuracy, and power. To achieve this, it helps us to be centered, grounded, and to think clearly. When we speak to someone, they may or may not truly listen. However, we can speak in a way that makes it more likely that they will hear. Regardless, we experience the joy that is earned when we speak the truth from a place of courage and integrity.

### OCCASIONS FOR USE

To be clear about the truth in a particular situation.

To help release emotions or thoughts that could interfere with communication, such as anger or fear.

To help us speak calmly and diplomatically.

### ENERGY CENTERS

General: Calms. Balances emotions.

Fifth: Supports the calm, clear speaking of truth.

### PHYSICAL SITES

Solar plexus, throat, buttocks, spine, shoulders.

### BLESSINGS

May I speak calmly and truthfully.

May I release all that interferes with communicating the truth effectively.

May I communicate without blame or judgement.

## AFFIRMATIONS

I perceive and speak the truth.

I have the courage to speak the truth.

I embrace discernment and release judgement.

## CHAMOMILE, ROMAN *(Anthemis nobilis)* FLOWERING PLANT
### FRANCE

## SPIRITUAL TEACHINGS

An old saying teaches that there is one mountain and many paths leading up that mountain. This illustrates the different ways people look for the sacred as well as honor Spirit. Roman Chamomile assists us in hearing both the holy voice and our inner voice in order to discern our individual path. Whether religious, or teachings that seem more secular such as art, this oil helps us to receive the teachings that have the most meaning for us and that speak most directly to who we are.

As we are assisted in finding our path, Roman Chamomile helps us to communicate our spiritual experience in a way that is not disrespectful of other paths. It helps us to speak in terms of celebrating all the spiritual journeys up the holy mountain. As we become more attuned to our personal journey and are able to tell others about it, Roman Chamomile calms and balances us so we can accept the limitations of being human, becoming more patient with ourselves.

## OCCASIONS FOR USE

To help us find our spiritual path.

When we are confused about our spiritual values.

To help us speak to others about our spiritual perspective.

To become more patient with our mistakes and setbacks on our spiritual path.

## ENERGY CENTERS

General: Calms. Balances emotions.

Seventh and Fifth: Connects these centers to facilitate hearing and communicating our spiritual truth.

Fourth: Eases grief and sadness.

Third: Helps us accept our limitations. Promotes patience. Eases tensions such as frustration and anger caused by the ego.

## PHYSICAL SITES

Temples, throat, middle back, liver, lungs.

## BLESSINGS

May I find my way up the mountain.

May I become more patient with myself as Spirit is patient with me.

May I know and speak the truth of Spirit.

May I speak of my spiritual path in such a way that it supports, encourages, and inspires others.

## AFFIRMATIONS

I listen to others with an open mind and heart.

I am clear about my spiritual path.

I am patient with my spiritual growth.


## CHAMPACA *(Michelia champaca)* BLOSSOMS

### INDIA

## SPIRITUAL TEACHINGS

Champaca develops intuition to help us "see" more clearly, in service to our spiritual growth. It gently persuades the ego (personality) to step aside so that we are more available to receive intuitive information for our highest good, rather than for serving and strengthening the ego. Champaca also assists us in being more receptive to the information that our spiritual guides are conveying to us. A unique aspect of this oil is that it helps us to stay grounded and in tune with our innate wisdom in such a way that we can discern which guide and which guidance will be most useful in a given situation. It helps us to know what to heed, as well as how to integrate the advice we receive.

OCCASIONS FOR USE

To help make a decision.

To receive the clearest and most helpful information about a situation.

To develop our intuition.

For assistance on our spiritual path.

To help balance our ego with our spirituality.

ENERGY CENTERS

General: Energizes and balances the subtle bodies and energy centers.

Seventh, Sixth, Fifth, Fourth, Third: Promotes higher levels of spiritual development.

Sixth: Helps us to be receptive to the Divine. Assists intuitive development.

PHYSICAL SITES

Base of skull, temples, ears, spine, solar plexus.

BLESSINGS

May I receive the information that serves my highest good and the highest good of all.

May I open to my intuitive abilities, and may they be in service to Spirit.

May I draw Spirit into my mind, heart, and body.

AFFIRMATIONS

I receive only the highest and most appropriate guidance.

I stand in grounded wisdom.

I place all my intuitive gifts in service to Spirit.

# CLARY SAGE *(Salvia sclarea)* FLOWERING PLANT

### BULGARIA

## SPIRITUAL TEACHINGS

Clary Sage strengthens the ability to dream and assists in the development of the intuitive mind, helping us access hidden truths and insights about others, ourselves, and our life experiences. Dreams can be a source of great teachings, offering an avenue to heal and grow, and even to solve our problems. Contemporary psychology values dreams as a way to understand the unconscious mind, and therapists may suggest that a client record her or his dreams or try to dream about a particular life issue as a way to understand it.

## OCCASIONS FOR USE

To help us remember our dreams.
To help us dream about a particular topic.
To help develop intuition.

## ENERGY CENTERS

General: Calms and uplifts.
Sixth: Increases dreaming. Supports our intuition to "see" more clearly. Inspires.

## PHYSICAL SITES

Temples, center of forehead, top of head, feet, lower stomach.

## BLESSINGS

May I be open to the wisdom and richness of dreaming.
May I honor my dreams as unique teachings.
May my intuition assist me in my spiritual growth.

## AFFIRMATIONS

I remember and heed my dreams.

The meanings of my dreams are clear to me.
I trust my intuition.

## COPAIVA BALM *(Copaifera reticulata)* RESIN
### BRAZIL

### SPIRITUAL TEACHINGS
In many traditions, the conscious, active mind is considered an obstacle to spirituality because it pulls us away from focusing on what is truly important. Copaiva balm brings discernment, helping us to concentrate on what is truly meaningful from a spiritual perspective. It also helps us to be more effective in dealing with the less important aspects of our lives. When our mind is aligned with the Divine, the gifts of vision, faith, humility, and wisdom are bestowed.

### OCCASIONS FOR USE
During times of mental stress and confusion.
To identify or reconnect with our spiritual goals.
To help us focus on what is spiritually important.
When we are spending too much time thinking about the future or reviewing the past.
To give us wisdom in a particular situation.

### ENERGY CENTERS
Seventh and Sixth: Connects these two centers, aligning the human mind with the
spiritual mind.

### PHYSICAL SITES
Top of head, center of forehead, feet.

### BLESSINGS
May I be focused and attuned to the Divine.

May I be wise in my thoughts and actions.
May I spend more time on what is truly important.

AFFIRMATIONS
My mind is aligned with Spirit.
I see clearly, and I focus on what is most important.


# CORIANDER *(Coriandrum sativum)* FRUIT

CROATIA / RUSSIA

## SPIRITUAL TEACHINGS
The field of body/mind/spirit medicine teaches us that our beliefs and thoughts affect our health—contributing to or impeding the healing process. In times of ill health, our beliefs about the nature of the illness, the reason for it, how long it will last, and the likely outcome have great influence. The specific gift of Coriander is to increase our confidence about the timing of healing. When we are open to the possibility of a more rapid recovery, our focused intention and belief in ourselves can make a real difference.

## OCCASIONS FOR USE
To assist in recovering from illness, whether it is physical or emotional.
When we are feeling depressed or unsure about our ability to heal.

## ENERGY CENTERS
General: Speeds the healing process.
Sixth: Improves memory.
Third: Promotes confidence and motivation.
Second: Increases creativity, spontaneity, and passion.
First: Promotes feelings of security.

PHYSICAL SITES
The location of the physical symptoms or illness, such as the head for a headache, the back for a backache, or the chest for a cough.

BLESSINGS
May I heal quickly and fully.
May my intention for healing align with Spirit.

AFFIRMATIONS
I am open to the right timing of healing.
I am ready to heal now.

# CYPRESS *(Cupressus sempervirens)* TWIGS
SPAIN

SPIRITUAL TEACHINGS
Perhaps one of the most profound and subtle teachings on the spiritual path is that "the path is the goal." It is the process—filled with lessons and change—not simply the end result that is important. Each step we take and each new transition furthers our journey. Life is filled with transitions, and Cypress will assist with any and all of these, but its gifts are most fully expressed in the transitions that accompany the spiritual path. Cypress helps us to have the courage to surrender our will to a higher purpose—to change, heal, transform, and go through the many deaths that accompany the birth of wisdom.

OCCASIONS FOR USE
To give us courage and patience during any type of change.
To help us surrender on our spiritual path.

ENERGY CENTERS

General: Strengthens and comforts. Assists in times of transition. Supports willing-
ness to change and transform.

Sixth: Promotes wisdom.

Third: Promotes confidence and patience.

PHYSICAL SITES

Spine, senses, hands, hips, feet.

BLESSINGS

May I be filled with patience and courage during this time of transition.

With each step, may I be closer to Spirit.

AFFIRMATIONS

I am ready and willing to change in service to my spiritual path.

I am strong and confident during this time of change.

ELEMI *(Canarium luzonicum)* RESIN

PHILLIPPINES

SPIRITUAL TEACHINGS:

The ancient alchemist, Hermes Trismegistus, wrote, "As above, so below." This recognition of the interconnectedness of all things is a foundational tenet of many mystical
and esoteric traditions. It declares that every event is meaningful, and that spirit and
matter are perfect reflections of one another.

Elemi is traditionally used in assisting people to ground after meditation. Its deeper
gift resides in understanding that what we do in the material world affects our spirit,
and that our spirit directly influences and impacts our experiences in the material
world. Elemi helps us find our place in the universe, teaching us to look for meaning

in every event of our lives and helping us to transform the most mundane into an expression of Spirit.

## OCCASIONS FOR USE

To ground before, during, and after meditation.

When life seems meaningless or mundane.

When spirituality seems very distant from daily life.

## ENERGY CENTERS

Seventh and Sixth: Opens us to mystical experiences. Deeply connects us to the Divine. Helps to balance our spiritual and worldly life.

First: Grounds after deep meditation. Balances the spiritual and worldly life.

## PHYSICAL SITES

Feet, temples, base of skull, solar plexus, hands, lower stomach.

## BLESSINGS

May I integrate the spiritual and material worlds in my life.

May I offer each moment, each thought, each feeling, and each action to the Divine.

## AFFIRMATIONS

I am a co-creator of all that I experience.

My life is a reflection of Spirit.

I am grounded in Earth and in Spirit.

## ERIGERON *(Coniza canadensis)* FLOWERING PLANT

### CANADA

## SPIRITUAL TEACHINGS

Our life purpose can be defined by what we do that gives us a sense of significance. "I am here to fight for justice by being a lawyer"; "My purpose is to be a good husband and father"; "I am here to teach"; these are examples of life-purpose statements. Many things can reflect our life purpose such as work, hobbies, interests, relationships, and spirituality.

When we are unsure about our purpose or feel we are going in the wrong direction, unhappiness can underlie a life that might appear successful on the outside, but feels empty or unsatisfying on the inside. Erigeron helps us to become clear about our life purpose, especially spiritually. It teaches us to listen to spiritual guidance as it directs us toward our most authentic life. When we are on our path, we are blessed with joy and satisfaction, even in the midst of difficult situations.

OCCASIONS FOR USE
When feeling unsure about one's life purpose.
When feeling empty and lost.
During times of transition, when life's purpose/path may be changing.

ENERGY CENTERS
General: Helps in discovering one's life purpose.
Seventh and Sixth: Opens these centers to receive spiritual guidance.

PHYSICAL SITES
Base of skull, spine, hips, buttocks, joints, feet, solar plexus.

BLESSINGS
May I know and walk my true path.
Show me my path and guide me in the steps.
May I know that I am worthy of, and able to fulfill, my life's purpose.

AFFIRMATIONS
I am open to discovering my true path.
I am ready to be who I am, and accomplish what I am intended to.
I am true to my deepest and highest self and purpose.

# EUCALYPTUS  *(Eucalyptus globulus* or *radiata)*  LEAVES
AUSTRALIA

## SPIRITUAL TEACHINGS

With today's fast-paced, complex lifestyles filled with responsibilities, it is common to feel exhausted and overwhelmed, as well as angry and frustrated. When this type of stress stays with us for too long without changing, it can cause both physical and emotional disharmony. Eucalyptus makes us aware of strong emotions associated with burn-out and stress, especially anger, and helps us to understand their purpose. It gently removes emotional energy blockages and helps us stop, take a deep breath, get a new perspective, and prioritize.

## OCCASIONS FOR USE

When we feel angry, frustrated, overwhelmed.

When strong negative emotions have been with us too long.

When we need help to prioritize.

To relieve stress associated with too many responsibilities.

## ENERGY CENTERS

General: Clears and cleanses a room. Dissolves energy blockages. Balances emotions.

Sixth: Inspires. Promotes concentration.

Fourth: Promotes room to breathe when feeling disheartened and suffocated
    by responsibilities.

## PHYSICAL SITES

Liver, knee, throat, base of skull, heart.

## BLESSINGS

May these negative emotions dissolve and flow away.

Help me prioritize and let go of what no longer serves me.

Help me to breathe and to clear away unnecessary responsibilities.

AFFIRMATIONS

I release all negative emotions that cause disharmony.

I choose a life that is balanced.

I can easily and effortlessly prioritize.

## FENNEL *(Foeniculum vulgare)* SEEDS
CROATIA

SPIRITUAL TEACHINGS

Learning to speak compassionately, appropriately, and truthfully is a primary precept and moral teaching on the spiritual path. Words have great power to harm or benefit others. Fennel aids the development of direct, authentic, and skillful communication. It helps us discover what we want to say, and then accurately express it to others in a positive way. Fennel also protects us from being harmed by someone else's negative words, as well as thoughts and deeds.

OCCASIONS FOR USE

To speak up in a situation that is uncomfortable for us.

To express ourselves authentically.

To help us communicate effectively.

To provide protection from negativity in uncomfortable situations.

ENERGY CENTERS

General: Provides protection from negative influences.

Fifth: Promotes authentic communication.

Third: Increases courage, confidence, and motivation.

PHYSICAL SITES

Throat, solar plexus, feet, buttocks.

## BLESSINGS

May I speak positively and compassionately.

May I be protected from the unkind words or deeds of another.

May I never harm another with my words.

## AFFIRMATIONS

I am protected and safe from negativity.

I am an effective, skillful, and truthful communicator.

## FIR, SILVER *(Abies alba)* CONES

AUSTRIA

## SPIRITUAL TEACHINGS

Emotions, both positive and negative, are ever-present on life's path as well as the spiritual path. When negative emotions such as fear, anger, or jealousy move through us, they can be catalysts for personal development and transformation. However, when they become stagnant, unfelt, and unprocessed, they block our energy and personal growth. Silver Fir teaches us to release energy blocks caused by unbalanced emotions—emotions unresolved from the past or unfelt in the present—without reliving them. This allows us to experience the power, integrity, and knowledge that are inherent in resolved emotions.

## OCCASIONS FOR USE

When strong emotions are making us feel ungrounded.

When our emotions are blocked because we cannot access our feelings, or cannot release them.

When we are afraid of what we are feeling.

## ENERGY CENTERS

General: Releases energy blocks. Balances emotions.

Sixth: Increases intuition.
First: Grounds.

## PHYSICAL SITES

Knees, feet, heart, pulse points, organ related to appropriate emotion (e.g. liver-
anger, lungs-grief).

## BLESSINGS

May I experience my true feelings.
May I learn from all of my emotions.
May I release all feelings that are ready to be released.

## AFFIRMATIONS

I honor my emotions.
I am strong, powerful, and secure in my emotions.

## FRANGIPANI *(Plumeria rubra)* BLOSSOMS

INDIA

## SPIRITUAL TEACHINGS

Some people on a spiritual path believe that the Earth is not spiritual, that earthly
experiences take us away from Spirit, and that the spiritual plane is superior to the
material plane. This leads to great personal suffering, for rejecting Earth and its physical nature means rejecting ourselves.

Frangipani connects us with the feminine nature of Earth—the mother and the
nurturer—whether we experience that essence as Mother Earth, Divine Mother, or
the feminine aspect of God. It teaches us that the material world, and every moment
on Earth, is infused with Spirit, and that leading a spiritual life must incorporate honoring and loving the earthly experience.

OCCASIONS FOR USE

When we feel disconnected from and/or superior to ordinary life.

When we feel distaste for the earthly experience.

When we want to remember and integrate Spirit in every moment.

ENERGY CENTERS

General: Promotes healing in our relationship with our Mother. Helps us expand
    our capacity to nurture others.

Seventh: Promotes an awareness of the feminine aspect of the Divine.

First: Helps to heal our relationship with Mother Earth. Helps spiritually focused
    people embrace and love the earthly experience.

PHYSICAL SITES

Left side of body, breasts, heart, upper back, lower stomach, feet.

BLESSINGS

May I walk lightly and lovingly upon this Earth.

May I honor Mother Earth in my heart, in my thoughts, and in every action and word.

Divine Mother, fill me with your compassion and grace.

AFFIRMATIONS

I embrace and honor the Earth.

My humanity is sacred.


## FRANKINCENSE *(Boswellia carterii)* RESIN

ETHIOPIA

SPIRITUAL TEACHINGS

The word for "breath" also means "spirit" or "life force" in several languages, and it symbolizes filling one with life. Breath is a perfect example of how Spirit infuses and merges

with matter, always and everywhere. Many traditions teach breathing meditation, in which focusing on the breath becomes a tool to clear the mind and expand consciousness.

Frankincense deepens our breath, calms and focuses our mind, and opens our consciousness to make clear, direct contact with the Divine. It has long been recognized as a sacred essential oil that helps to heal the spirit and comfort the heart. It creates a mindful, meditative state in which we can experience and integrate Divine wisdom. Frankincense teaches us that peace, enlightenment, healing, and wisdom are ever-present—just a breath away.

OCCASIONS FOR USE
To ground and open consciousness, and to connect with the Divine
    during meditation.
To connect body, mind, and spirit on the spiritual path.
To help in pursuit of enlightenment and grace.

ENERGY CENTERS
General: Calms, comforts, and centers. Stabilizes emotions.
Seventh: Focuses and strengthens spiritual consciousness and enlightenment.
    Connects us with the eternal and Divine.
Sixth: Quiets and clarifies the mind. Promotes a meditative state.
First: Grounds.

PHYSICAL SITES
Top of head, temples, feet, length of back.

BLESSINGS
May each breath be a prayer.
Spirit, fill and bless me as I breathe.

AFFIRMATIONS
My mind is quiet and calm.

I focus on my breath.

I am at peace.

## GERANIUM *(Pelargonium graveolens* or *roseum)* FLOWERING PLANT
### REUNION OR CHINA

### SPIRITUAL TEACHINGS

Many of us complain about not having enough time—our lives can be so frantically busy that we are unable to find moments of stillness and relaxation. Overwhelmed by too much to do, we are impaired in our ability to nurture our creativity, our relationships, and our connection with body/mind/spirit. The faster we go, the more quality time we lose.

Geranium is a profoundly feminine oil that helps us create and identify what truly nurtures and sustains us. It helps us to relax and to calm our body, mind, and spirit so that we can connect with ourselves, other people, and the environment around us. Able to balance stillness and movement, and spontaneity and structure, it also helps draw toward us what we need. Like the fallow soil of winter bursting forth with the extraordinary life of spring, Geranium creates a quiet, balanced place where life emerges naturally, creatively, and joyfully.

### OCCASIONS FOR USE

When feeling frantic from being too busy.

To be more creative.

To help discipline ourselves in service to the life we want and need.

### ENERGY CENTERS

General: Calms the mind and spirit. Promotes harmony and happiness in relationships. Balances the emotions.

Seventh and Sixth: Balances the mind and spirit. Provides spiritual protection.

Fifth: Increases the capacity for intimate communication.

Third: Helps us to gain control over our lives.

Second: Fosters creativity. Nourishes feminine creativity. Promotes relaxed spontaneity.

## PHYSICAL SITES

Temples, throat, hands, shoulders.

## BLESSINGS

May I be blessed with the sweetness of silence.

Help me create the life that most truly sustains me.

May I slow my pace to enjoy life more fully.

## AFFIRMATIONS

I create the time to relax, meditate, and discover what I truly need and want.

I create the time to nurture my relationships.

I am balanced in mind and spirit.

## GINGER *(Zingiber officinalis)* RHIZOME
### VIETNAM

## SPIRITUAL TEACHINGS

The experience of abundance begins with gratitude—for our life and all that we have. If we are appreciative, we create the space and capability to manifest our desires, drawing them to us. Ginger strengthens us on all levels so that we have the courage and confidence to identify what we want, and then to create it. It invites abundance, helping us tap into the extraordinary richness of the universe. It also helps us believe that we deserve to experience abundant life.

## OCCASIONS FOR USE

When we want to bring something specific into our lives.

When we want to experience gratitude or the sense of abundance.
When we want to build confidence about manifesting and drawing what we
   want to us.

ENERGY CENTERS
General: Strengthens.
Third: Promotes courage and confidence.
Second: Increases sexual desire.
First: Attracts prosperity.

PHYSICAL SITES
Pulse points, feet, palms of hands, shoulders, lower back.

BLESSINGS
May the abundance of the universe flow through me.
May I be ever grateful for all I have.

AFFIRMATIONS
I am deserving.
I am confident and able to create what I want in life.
I am ready to experience _____ in my life.


## GUAIAC WOOD *(Bulnesia sarmienti)* WOOD
**BRAZIL**

SPIRITUAL TEACHINGS
Guaiac Wood allows the personal will to enter into a true relationship with Divine will, helping the entire personality to develop spiritually. It aligns the personal will and personality with Divine will and guidance. It teaches us about the integrity of the personality as a vehicle for spirituality in the world. It blesses us with healthy humility, balanced power, and clarity.

OCCASIONS FOR USE

During times of power struggles with others.

When our ego is out of balance with our spiritual path.

When we need clarity about our spirituality.

ENERGY CENTERS

Seventh and Third: Encourages spirituality to influence personal will. Helps prepare
the personality for spiritual development.

PHYSICAL SITES

Lower stomach, hands, shoulders, temples, buttocks.

BLESSINGS

Thy will be done.

May my actions be in balance with Spirit.

Make me an instrument of thy will.

AFFIRMATIONS

My personality is a vehicle for my highest purpose.

My will is aligned with Divine will and guidance.


GURJUM    *(Dipterocarpus turbinatua)*    RESIN

INDONESIA

SPIRITUAL TEACHINGS

Gurjum teaches us that intuitive, contemplative exercises for the mind help us connect with our spiritual source and sustenance, as well as access states of consciousness
that open the mind to spiritual information. It also balances intuition with the higher
self, helping them work well together. Gurjum reminds us that Spirit can speak to us
through our intuition, and that taking the time to meditate or pray invites the spiritual realm into our consciousness and therefore our life.

OCCASIONS FOR USE

To help us begin a spiritual practice of meditation or prayer.

To help us develop our intuition.

When feeling spiritually depleted or disconnected.

ENERGY CENTERS

General: Supports meditative states. Activates the intuitive mind.

Seventh and Sixth: Helps to open these centers to receive spiritual energy.

PHYSICAL SITES

Temples, top of head, base of skull, feet.

BLESSINGS

May I always hear the words of Spirit.

May I receive the love and wisdom of the sacred.

May I be refreshed and replenished.

AFFIRMATIONS

I use my intuition for the highest good.

I trust my intuition.

I am committed to my spiritual practice.

## HAY *(Foenum)* PLANT

FRANCE

SPIRITUAL TEACHINGS

Spiritual lessons and guidance have many origins, such as people, angels, animals, and plants, all aiming to help us become balanced in body, mind, and spirit. We all have guardian angels, special animals, and plants that particularly resonate with who we are and assist us in times of need. Indeed, this entire book is about being attuned to the teachings and the wisdom of the plant kingdom as it is distilled into essential oils. Hay will help you to hear, understand, and heed the teachings of plants and the role they can play in your spiritual growth.

OCCASIONS FOR USE

To connect with the teachings of plants.

To connect with nature in a grounded and spiritual way.

When we are studying herbology, aromatherapy, or flower essences.

When we are planting or tending a garden.

ENERGY CENTERS

General: Assists with meditation. Helps connect with intuitive guidance, especially from the plant kingdom.

PHYSICAL SITES

Feet, temples.

BLESSINGS

May I hear and integrate the teachings of plants.

Bless the plant kingdom and its wisdom.

AFFIRMATIONS

I honor the life force in every plant.

I am open to the teaching of the plant kingdom.


IMMORTELLE *(Helichrysum italicum* or *angustifolium)* FLOWERING PLANT

FRANCE/CROATIA

SPIRITUAL TEACHINGS

We all have intuitive abilities, and there are times when we want to share with others what we have perceived. On the spiritual path, it is important that the information is conveyed with respect, empathy, and in a compassionate manner. When our hearts and intuition are in tune, they allow us to be in relationship with both guidance and another person. In this way, it is more likely that the information will be received and truly useful.

Immortelle activates and supports the intuitive mind. It also helps to integrate the heart with Spirit, so that the information you perceive can be shared in gentle and loving service to others. It helps us discern when to share our perceptions, and when to keep them to ourselves. This powerful essential oil grounds us in Divine love and guidance, fostering understanding and compassionate insight.

OCCASIONS FOR USE
To access our intuitive abilities.
To develop compassion for and understanding of oneself and others.
To know if, when, and how to share our intuitive insights with others.

ENERGY CENTERS
General: Dissolves energy blocks. Balances the upper energy centers.
Sixth: Activates the right side of the brain (intuitive/creative). Assists in communicating intuitive impressions. Promotes understanding.
Fourth: Promotes compassion for self and others. Integrates compassion and spirituality.

PHYSICAL SITES
Temples, throat, center of forehead, heart, solar plexus.

BLESSINGS
May my heart and mind be as one.
May I be filled with compassion.
May I speak all that I perceive in the most compassionate manner.
May I know when and how to share my perceptions.

AFFIRMATIONS
I speak my impressions, free of blame and judgement, from a place of compassion.

My intuition is aligned with my heart and Spirit.
I speak only when it is for the highest good.


## JASMINE  *(Jasminum officinale)* BLOSSOMS
### INDIA

### SPIRITUAL TEACHINGS

The Chinese yin/yang symbol elegantly illustrates the spiritual teaching that opposites comprise a whole, and that within each component there is a seed of the other. In our everyday reality, we may believe that we must be or choose in an either/or manner—either masculine or feminine, introverted or extroverted, happy or sad, successful or a failure, spiritual or secular.

Jasmine helps us identify the illusionary opposites. There are situations that demand a choice, but Jasmine shows us where "either/or" can be expanded into "both/and." One of the primary cultural and spiritual separations addressed by Jasmine is that between love and sexuality. Jasmine blesses and blends both, acquainting sexuality with the sweetness of real love, and helping love to passionately, safely, and honestly express itself in the intimacy of sexuality. It is a profoundly feminine oil that embraces and exults the sacred masculine.

### OCCASIONS FOR USE

When love and sex are separated in our hearts and minds.
To help us develop a broader perspective.
To help us understand the contradictions in our lives.

### ENERGY CENTERS

General: Unites and harmonizes opposites to promote wholeness. Calms, soothes, relaxes, and lifts the spirits. Releases worry to allow living in the present moment.
Seventh: Connects spirituality and sexuality. Heightens spiritual awareness.

Sixth: Enhances intuition. Opens the mind to deeper truths. Inspires.

Fourth: Warms and opens the heart.

Second: Promotes love and sensuality. Connects spirituality and sexuality. Promotes creativity and artistic development.

## PHYSICAL SITES

Breasts, heart, base of skull, pulse points, lower stomach.

## BLESSINGS

May I understand and embrace a broad perspective.

May the dualities in my life be as one.

Bless my sexuality.

## AFFIRMATIONS

I embrace and enfold all duality.

I honor the feminine and masculine in others and myself.

I celebrate my sexuality.

## JUNIPER *(Juniperus communis)* BERRIES

CROATIA

## SPIRITUAL TEACHINGS

Juniper clears our body/mind/spirit of the damaging perceptions that interfere with our confidence and sense of self-worth. It releases old thoughts, strengthens our intuition, and deepens trust in our inner voice. Juniper teaches that a clear mind prepares us to listen to Spirit and integrate what we have heard. Juniper is also one of the primary oils to protect us from the negativity of others, and it helps to release anything that has already affected us. Through this energetic detoxification, we are free to grow in spiritual wisdom.

## OCCASIONS FOR USE

To release outmoded thoughts and beliefs.

To become more confident.

To help us grow in wisdom.

To release any negativity we have accepted from others.

To protect ourselves energetically when we are in a situation that is challenging or in some way potentially harmful for us.

## ENERGY CENTERS

General: Clears and cleanses a room of negative energies. Protects against negative influences. Clears energetic blockages. Cleanses and detoxifies the subtle bodies.

Seventh: Helps us to connect with and act from our highest ideals. Enlightens.

Sixth: Dispels mental stagnation. Assists clairvoyance if used for altruistic reasons. Promotes inner vision and wisdom.

Third: Strengthens will power and eases fear of failure, restoring confidence and increasing self-worth.

## PHYSICAL SITES

Center of forehead, solar plexus, crown of head, buttocks, lower stomach.

## BLESSINGS

May I open my mind to the Divine.

May I release all negativity that I have accepted—consciously and unconsciously.

Help me to be confident and secure in myself.

May I listen to and hear my inner voice.

## AFFIRMATIONS

I release all outmoded thoughts that interfere with my self-worth.

I act with clarity and wisdom.

I am protected from the negativity of others.

## LAVENDER *(Lavendula vera)* FLOWERING PLANT
FRANCE

### SPIRITUAL TEACHINGS

The Navajo people's Beauty Way teaches that a spiritual life is one in which we walk in balance on the Earth. This means being attuned to the environment like a dancer is attuned to his or her partner; being awake and attentive like a martial artist who moves when necessary and is still when needed. Few people can live at all times from this place of balance, but it is a worthy goal for all of us. Perhaps our task is simply to be as present as possible in each moment.

Lavender, an exquisite yet common essential oil, teaches us to be balanced and to live in the present, on all levels—physical, emotional, mental, and spiritual. When we are depleted, it energizes. When we are anxious, it calms and relaxes. Lavender shows us the balance point in each moment. It also helps us to release whatever interferes with the present. Lavender is a true escort on the path of the Beauty Way.

### OCCASIONS FOR USE

When we are feeling unbalanced in any way.
To increase self-awareness.
To release negativity or anything preventing us from being present.
To help us relax when we are feeling anxious and tense.

### ENERGY CENTERS

General: Clears and cleanses a room. Brings in positive energy. Balances all centers and subtle bodies.
Seventh: Helps to integrate spirituality in everyday life. Promotes spiritual growth.
Fourth: Calms, comforts, and stabilizes emotions of the heart. Promotes compassion.

### PHYSICAL SITES

Top of head, center of forehead, heart, feet, hips, knees, hands, any site experiencing pain or discomfort.

BLESSINGS

May I be present and balanced.

May I be a source of blessing and healing for others.

May I walk in beauty.

Iroquois night chant: May beauty be before me, may beauty be behind me. May beauty be to my right and to my left. May beauty be above me, may beauty be below me, may beauty be all around me. In beauty it is finished. HO.

AFFIRMATIONS

I walk in balance on this Earth.

I am relaxed, energized, and present.

I am a woman/man of beauty.

I am whole.


# LEMON *(Citrus limonum)* RIND
## URUGUAY

SPIRITUAL TEACHINGS

One of the challenges of using our intuition is to try to remain objective. We need to be sure that our personal issues, opinions, prejudices, and moods do not interfere too much, because they influence the information we receive. Even under the best of circumstances, intuition remains a human and therefore imperfect tool. Rosalyn Bruyere, an accomplished intuitive and healer, estimates that most intuitive people, on their best days, are about 85% accurate.

Lemon is a joyous, energizing essential oil that helps to open and strengthen our intuition. It encourages us to be more fully present, focused, and clear for intuitive impressions, helping us stay grounded in the heart and objective in the mind.

OCCASIONS FOR USE

To help receive and understand intuitive information.

When our emotions or thoughts are interfering with our intuition.

ENERGY CENTERS
General: Clears and cleanses a room. Clears emotional confusion. Energizes.
Sixth: Promotes objectivity and mental clarity. Focuses consciousness. Opens and
   strengthens intuition.
Fourth: Helps to alleviate fears of emotional involvement. Promotes joy.

PHYSICAL SITES
Center of forehead, base of skull, pulse points, solar plexus, feet.

BLESSINGS
May all that blocks my intuition be released.
May I be filled with joy.
May my mind be clear.
May I intuit the truth.

AFFIRMATIONS
I see the truth with clarity and objectivity.
I trust my intuition.
I am present and focused.

## LEPTOSPERMUM *(Leptospermum citratum)* LEAVES
NEW ZEALAND

SPIRITUAL TEACHINGS
As we acquaint ourselves with the spiritual teachings of indigenous people, we appreciate the ancient wisdom-teachings of the Earth. Native people know about seasonal
cycles and the invaluable lessons from animals, plants, stones, and Spirit.
Leptospermum helps those of us who live in the modern world to learn the profound

wisdom of these teachings. It helps us to understand them, integrate them, and apply them to the way in which we live now.

OCCASIONS FOR USE
To feel connected to the Earth.
When we are studying the teachings of indigenous peoples.
To feel aligned with the cycles of nature.
To help us understand the wisdom of animals and plants.

ENERGY CENTERS
Sixth: Helps us understand and integrate the ancient wisdom of indigenous people.

PHYSICAL SITES
Feet, heart, solar plexus, hands.

BLESSINGS
Bless the Earth and her teachings.
May I learn the wisdom of the Earth.

AFFIRMATIONS
I am open to the teaching of ancient peoples.
I honor the ancient teachings.
Earth, animals, and plants are my teachers.


## MANDARIN *(Citrus reticulata)* RIND
USA

SPIRITUAL TEACHINGS
It is not unusual for spiritual work and development to involve psychological issues. Wounds in the personality need to be tended so the personality can be more thor-

oughly infused with the Divine. Mandarin assists in connecting us with our inner child—the part of our character that developed early in life. It helps us heal and release unhappy events, as well as experience the joy and ebullience of childhood. Remembering the challenges of our early life can be uncomfortable, yet Mandarin helps us access the happiness as well. It inspires and encourages our rediscovery of the innocence and radiant joy within all of us.

## OCCASIONS FOR USE

When working on childhood issues.
To help us find the joyful child within.
To relate better with children.
To bring more playfulness and inspiration into our lives.

## ENERGY CENTERS

General: Promotes joy and happiness.
Sixth: Inspires.
Fifth: Promotes communication with the inner child.

## PHYSICAL SITES

Temples, pulse points, solar plexus, ankles.

## BLESSINGS

May I remember the happiness of my childhood.
May I experience the joy of childhood.
May I be filled with happiness and the innocent sweetness of a child.

## AFFIRMATIONS

I am energized and delighted by play.
I am willing and ready to remember, heal, and celebrate my inner child.

## MASTIC *(Pistacia lentiscus)* LEAVES / TWIGS
FRANCE

### SPIRITUAL TEACHINGS
The body is our physical vehicle on Earth, as well as the vessel for Spirit and spiritual information. Mastic supports and helps to strengthen and energize the body so it is better able to receive spiritual teachings and embody them. This oil will particularly help those people whose spiritual path is in service to others.

### OCCASIONS FOR USE
When we are physically exhausted, especially during times of giving.

To prevent and/or heal burn-out.

To strengthen the body/mind/spirit for doing service work. Mastic is especially good for providers of care such as nurses or therapists.

To help us demonstrate our spiritual beliefs through action.

### ENERGY CENTERS
Seventh: Creates a direct and immediate connection with Divine guidance.

Fourth: Balances the compassionate heart.

Second: Provides emotional protection.

First: Strengthens the physical body.

### PHYSICAL SITES
Heart, lower stomach, spine, shoulders, full back, pulse points.

### BLESSINGS
May I be an instrument of Divine love.

May I be strong in service to others.

May I be infused with physical vitality and grace of spirit.

## AFFIRMATIONS
My physical body is strong and capable.
I draw Divine energy into my body.
My body is a vehicle for Spirit.

## MELISSA *(Melissa officinalis)* PLANT
FRANCE

## SPIRITUAL TEACHINGS
Everyone must come to terms with the certainty of death. We cannot avoid the reality of experiencing grief. We search for meaning in the midst of loss. There are many ways of understanding death and loss, but inevitably we face a difficult spiritual task: to feel grief yet keep our hearts open and capable of giving and receiving. Melissa helps us release emotional blocks and heal the wounds caused by the death of a loved one. It teaches us that death is a part of life, without interfering in the natural grief process.

## OCCASIONS FOR USE
During times of grief.
When our heart feels constricted and unable to grieve.
When there has been a death of any kind—a person, a dream, a relationship, a job, or hope.

## ENERGY CENTERS
General: Helps one deal with issues surrounding death. Promotes emotional clarity. Promotes understanding and acceptance.
Seventh: Promotes spiritual growth.
Fourth: Relieves emotional blocks, especially due to grief.

## PHYSICAL SITES
Heart, temples, lungs, spine.

BLESSINGS

May my heart be strong, yet open.

May this grief pass.

Bless all endings and all new beginnings.

AFFIRMATIONS

I open my heart to grief, with love.

I am capable of loving and giving, despite this great loss.

I honor death as a part of life.

## MONARDA *(Monarda didyma)* FLOWERING PLANT

CANADA

SPIRITUAL TEACHINGS

Monarda is a gatekeeper and guardian of the spiritual path. It regulates the flow of spiritual information, and gently prepares the body and personality to be able to receive, integrate, and act upon the information received. It prepares us on all levels for the next step on our path, helping us to become new vessels into which the wine of compassionate wisdom can be poured. Monarda prevents the feeling of being overwhelmed. It teaches that steady, patient, and disciplined surrender opens us to Spirit and transforms us on a cellular level.

OCCASIONS FOR USE

To encourage spiritual lessons or, conversely, to slow them.

When needing support and validation for our current position on our spiritual path.

To appreciate the timing of our spiritual lessons.

To help our body and personality prepare for spiritual growth.

ENERGY CENTERS

Seventh: Allows us to perceive, receive, or understand information for which we are ready. Prevents spiritual confusion and overload. Assists the body and personality to prepare for spiritual growth and to gently integrate the spiritual information that is received.

## PHYSICAL SITES
Top of head, temples, base of skull, feet, shoulders, spine, joints.

## BLESSINGS
May I walk with grace, love, and intention on my spiritual path.
May I accept Divine timing, rather than my own.
May I be a balanced and blessed vessel for Divine love.
May my personality be gently healed to better represent Spirit.

## AFFIRMATIONS
I embrace the perfection of who I am right now.
I value each stage of my spiritual path.
My body and personality are healed and transformed.
I am prepared for spiritual truths.

## MYRRH *(Commiphora myrrha)* RESIN
SOMALIA

## SPIRITUAL TEACHINGS
There is a belief in many spiritual traditions that our greatest teachings are found within our emotional wounds. Our task is to accept life's challenges and allow them to teach us compassionate wisdom—a great spiritual gift that enables us to feel compassion for the suffering of others as well as ourselves. This does not mean that we should cling to our wounds, but rather use our healing to support and assist others.

Myrrh helps us get through the trials and tribulations of life. It helps us to understand and cope with our inevitable human, physical/emotional/psychological wounds.

It supports and protects us, gives us strength, and opens us intuitively so we can experience the presence of Spirit. Held and blessed by Myrrh, we have the capacity to face, feel, and integrate some of the most potent earthly challenges.

OCCASIONS FOR USE

When feeling exhausted or overwhelmed by our own troubles or the
    suffering of others.
To help us understand, from a spiritual perspective, the meaning of
    emotional challenges.

ENERGY CENTERS

General: Strengthens and energizes. Supports earthly manifestations of dreams and
    visions by linking higher energy centers with the base energy center.
Seventh: Assists us in moving forward on our spiritual journey. Fortifies spirituality.
Sixth and First: Grounds during meditation.
Fifth: Provides support for confident communication.
Fourth: Eases sorrow and grief.

PHYSICAL SITES

Heart, spine, shoulders, lower stomach, hips, throat, knees, feet, joints.

BLESSINGS

May I learn and grow from everything I experience.
May my suffering help me to be of service to others.
May my spirit be refreshed.
May I understand that all trials eventually pass.

AFFIRMATIONS

I am a compassionate witness to the pain and suffering of myself and others.
My wounds are my greatest teachers.
I accept the challenges of life.

## NEROLI *(Citrus aurantium)* BLOSSOMS
MOROCCO

### SPIRITUAL TEACHINGS

The Kahuna shamans of Hawaii teach that there are three aspects of the mind that relate to the manifestation of our goals and desires—the conscious mind, subconscious mind (soul), and super-conscious (spirit) mind. The conscious mind is the ordinary, day-to-day awareness in which we function in the present moment. This is where we formulate our goals. The subconscious mind holds all the hidden aspects of our psyche, such as our fears, our memories, and our beliefs about ourselves, other people, and the world. The super-conscious mind manifests, bringing our desires to reality.

The Hawaiian medicine people say that if we consciously decide to bring something into our lives, accompanied by ceremonies, prayers, and affirmation, it will manifest. If it does not, there is something in the subconscious creating a psychological block. Neroli is the essential oil that assists the subconscious mind to reveal itself and unite with the conscious mind, bringing awareness to the present moment and helping to resolve blocks. This releases a flood of positive energy that becomes available to the super-conscious. As this energy flows from self to soul to spirit, we are in direct communication with the world of manifestation. Neroli helps us manifest our deepest and highest aspirations.

### OCCASIONS FOR USE

To help us become aware of unresolved issues so we can deal with them.

To increase consciousness.

To attune more fully to our spiritual path.

To help us manifest our desires.

### ENERGY CENTERS

General: Brings in positive energy. Relaxes. Helps us face our emotional fears. Links lower and higher selves—soul and spirit.

Seventh: Promotes direct communication with the spiritual world.

Sixth: Reunites the conscious and subconscious mind.

Fourth: Eases grief. Helps us experience joyful love.

Third: Supports manifestation.

Second: Promotes sensual comfort.

## PHYSICAL SITES

Hands, temples, center of forehead, lower stomach, knees, feet, heart.

## BLESSINGS

May I walk with my spirit and soul aligned.

Help me to know and heal my unresolved issues.

Help me create what I truly desire.

## AFFIRMATIONS

I am ready to create new beliefs.

I am free of my past.

I release all that blocks my ability to manifest.


## OAKMOSS  *(Evernia prunastri)*  MOSS

CROATIA

## SPIRITUAL TEACHINGS

Oakmoss helps to ground us, deeply and securely, while healing past traumas that prevent us from being fully present. It gently allows us to release fear and mistrust, opening our heart to embrace physical experience—its joys as well as sorrows. When we are fully able to be in the here and now, we are opened to receiving the generosity and abundance of the earthly experience. For some people, this will be in the form of monetary wealth. For others, it will reveal itself as emotional, creative, resourceful, or inspirational abundance. Oakmoss promotes the types of abundance that will be most spiritually profound for the individual. It also helps to integrate the experience of true security that is not associated with money, possessions, or accomplishments—one that is founded on trusting the generosity and ultimate safety of the universe.

## OCCASIONS FOR USE

To be grounded and present in the body, in the moment.

To increase our experiences of abundance.

When we are uncertain about prosperity.

To ground during meditation.

To feel physically or emotionally safe and secure.

## ENERGY CENTERS

First: Increases a sense of safety, prosperity, and security. Promotes a sense of joy about being in a physical body.

## PHYSICAL SITES

Feet, lower stomach, palms of hands, solar plexus, pulse points.

## BLESSINGS

May I be grounded in the earthly experience as I walk on my spiritual path.

May I be nurtured and filled by the abundance of Mother Earth.

May I trust in the generosity of the universe.

## AFFIRMATIONS

I am grounded, protected, and safe.

I deserve prosperity.

I am emotionally comfortable and at peace.

## ORANGE *(Citrus aurantium)* RIND

USA

### SPIRITUAL TEACHINGS

People who meet the Dalai Lama often comment on the extraordinary joy that he radiates. His eyes are surrounded by fine laugh lines, his giggle is infectious, and even though he has experienced incredible suffering, his strength, compassion, serenity, and faith inspire all who meet him. Like the Dalai Lama, women and men who are masters on their spiritual path tend to radiate extraordinary joy and delight. Orange oil teaches us about that joy—the positive, courageous, creative energy that nourishes the soul, helping us become more confident and loving. We can face our challenges and embrace our experiences—all in the spirit of joy.

### OCCASIONS FOR USE

When feeling depressed.

When feeling lethargic.

When we lack confidence.

When we are physically, emotionally, intellectually, or spiritually depleted.

### ENERGY CENTERS

General: Brings in positive energy. Nourishes the soul with joy. Mobilizes stagnated energy.

Fourth: Promotes joyful love.

Third: Promotes self-confidence and courage.

Second: Promotes joy in sexuality and the creative process.

### PHYSICAL SITES

Heart, solar plexus, upper back, pulse points, knees.

BLESSINGS
May I be blessed with joy and filled with delight.
May I be a source of joy to others.
May I be courageous through life's experiences.

AFFIRMATIONS
I delight in the universe.
I am confident and creative.
I feel joy.

## PALMAROSA *(Cympobogon martinii)* FLOWERING PLANT
NEPAL

SPIRITUAL TEACHINGS
The word "healing" is derived from the Anglo-Saxon word *haelen,* which means "to make whole." Palmarosa supports the process of healing the body, mind, and spirit and helps prevent problems from recurring. It assists the breaking down, breaking through, and breaking forth that leads to wholeness. It also helps with the timing of healing so the process can be deeply and completely integrated into the body, mind, and spirit.

OCCASIONS FOR USE
During any kind of healing process, whether physical, psychological, or spiritual.
To help us be patient during a healing process.

ENERGY CENTERS
General: Aids in all types of healing—physical, emotional, mental, and spiritual.
Sixth: Clears the mind to help with decision-making. Develops wisdom.
Fourth: Comforts the heart.
First: Encourages feelings of security.

## PHYSICAL SITES
Wherever healing is needed. Examples: Lower back for lower back ache, temples for
   worry, heart for grief, top of head for feeling lost on one's spiritual path.

## BLESSINGS
May I be healed.
Fill me with your healing love.
Divine wholeness, heal me on all levels.

## AFFIRMATIONS
I am healed.
I am ready to heal.
I am balanced in body, mind, and spirit.

## PATCHOULI *(Pogostemon patchouli)* PLANT
INDONESIA

## SPIRITUAL TEACHINGS
Patchouli teaches that the physical body is sacred and that our senses are avenues to
our soul and doorways to Spirit. Patchouli asks us to experience our senses and sensuality as a sacred gift. It helps the mind to relax and connect with the knowledge of
the body. It reminds us that every act of creation—making a meal, writing a letter, giving birth to a child, or building a home—honors the original act of creation. Patchouli
is grounding yet enlightens our minds, and brings pleasure and delight.

## OCCASIONS FOR USE
When we believe that our sensuality is not spiritual.
When we are unable to be or feel creative.
When we are tense or worried.
When we want to sense the integration of body, mind, and spirit.

ENERGY CENTERS

General: Grounds and soothes.

Sixth: Relaxes a tense and overactive mind.

Second: Spiritualizes sexuality. Awakens creativity and the enjoyment of the senses.

First: Strengthens and grounds. Supports the connection of the physical body
    and the subtle bodies.

PHYSICAL SITES

Feet, lower stomach, lower back, temples.

BLESSINGS

May I be grounded in body, mind, and spirit.

May my creativity express the joy of Spirit.

May my senses teach me to play and celebrate with Spirit.

AFFIRMATIONS

I create in remembrance and celebration of all creation.

My creativity flows easily and joyfully.

My mind is calm and relaxed.


PINE  *(Pinus cembra* or *sylvestris)* NEEDLES

AUSTRIA / BULGARIA

SPIRITUAL TEACHINGS

We live in a culture that values high energy and high performance, but tends to ignore the body's natural rhythms and its need for sleep, rest, and replenishment. It is no wonder that so many people feel depleted physically, psychologically, and/or spiritually. From this place of exhaustion, we can be left feeling empty, even after all of our accomplishments. Pine's teachings are related to the Greek god Pan—the masculine archetypal symbol of the fertility, abundance, and playfulness of the natural world. Pan is joyful and exuberant, and in tune with the cycles of nature.

Pine energizes and helps the body, mind, and heart to replenish. It aligns the energy of the body and focus of the will, without force, so they work together as a team—the body responding to the will's direction, and the will honoring the body's need for rest, work, and play. Pine clears away feelings of being emotionally or spiritually stagnant and fills us with delight, purpose, and vitality.

OCCASIONS FOR USE
To restore self-confidence and will.
When we are feeling depleted—physically, emotionally, mentally, spiritually.
When we lack feelings of joy and enthusiasm.

ENERGY CENTERS
Third: Energizes. Clarifies personal will. Dispels negativity.
Second: Promotes creativity, playfulness, sensuality.

PHYSICAL SITES
Lower stomach, solar plexus, palms of hands, hips, joints, ankles, feet.

BLESSINGS
May I be filled with the energy of nature.
May I be in tune with my natural rhythms.
May I move forward on my spiritual path with energy and joy.

AFFIRMATIONS
I have all the energy I need.
My mind, will, and body are rejuvenated and aligned.
I am filled with exuberance and delight.

## ROSE *(Rosa centifolia* or *damascena)* BLOSSOMS
### MOROCCO / BULGARIA

### SPIRITUAL TEACHINGS

For many people on a spiritual path, love and compassionate wisdom are the greatest teachings. Rose is the oil that teaches the lessons of love. It has been said that the universe is the overflow and outpouring of Spirit's ebullient love. Sacred to the Divine feminine and the angelic realm, the extraordinary energy of Rose assists us in healing our emotional wounds so we can better give and receive love, unconditionally. It helps us to heal the pain caused by grief and teaches us how to forgive others when they have hurt us. It surrounds us with the aroma of beauty so that our heart can open, heal, and blossom. Rose also gently seals and protects our energy field so that we are not affected by negativity.

### OCCASIONS FOR USE

When our heart is aching due to any kind of emotional pain.

When we feel hurt by others.

To forgive others as well as ourselves.

To learn how to be more loving and compassionate.

When we are feeling depressed, lonely, or disconnected.

### ENERGY CENTERS

General: Brings in positive energy. Gently fills holes in the energy field and seals it to protect us. Promotes a sense of well-being.

Seventh: Promotes a sense of spiritual connection and completeness.

Fourth: Promotes love, compassion, hope, and patience. Calms and supports. Heals emotional wounds, especially grief.

Second: Connects sexuality with the heart center. Promotes creativity and love of beauty.

Hands: Energetically connects the hands to the heart.

## PHYSICAL SITES
Heart, lower stomach, temples, lungs, knees, hands.

## BLESSINGS
May I learn to be more loving.
May I be more compassionate to those around me.
May I be an instrument of God's love.
May my emotional wounds be healed.

## AFFIRMATIONS
My heart is healed.
I am lovable.
I am a loving person.
I give and receive love.

## ROSEMARY *(Rosmarinus officinalis)* FLOWERING PLANT
SPAIN

## SPIRITUAL TEACHINGS
When asked what the monks do in the monastery, a Buddhist monk once replied with a smile, "We remember, and forget, and remember and forget, and remember." This humorously reminds us that no matter how attentive we are to our spiritual life, in the midst of daily chores and challenges we can lose our focus, forgetting that our relationship with Spirit is the most important thing in our life.

Rosemary teaches us to tend to our spiritual path in several important ways. It promotes mental clarity, helping us remember what we truly value. It helps us create and maintain healthy boundaries in relationships, so we do not lose ourselves to others. It strengthens our relationship with Spirit and fortifies our will power so we can walk our spiritual path with purpose and intent. Lastly, Rosemary deepens our joyful, loving connection with the sustenance of faith and the tender, powerful truth that we are always with Spirit.

## OCCASIONS FOR USE
To help promote mental, emotional, and spiritual clarity.
To help us have appropriate and healthy boundaries with others.
To develop self-confidence and will.
To deepen and strengthen our faith.
To help us remember our spiritual path and values.

## ENERGY CENTERS
General: Clears and cleanses a room. Provides protection from negative influences. Helps to establish healthy boundaries in relationships. Strengthens and centers.
Seventh: Helps us to strengthen our spiritual path. Inspires faith.
Sixth: Clears the mind. Enhances memory. Promotes clear thoughts, insights, and understanding.
Fourth: Inspires joyful love.
Third: Promotes self-confidence. Promotes action. Strengthens will power.

## PHYSICAL SITES
Temples, top of head, center of forehead, solar plexus, lower stomach.

## BLESSINGS
May I remember what is most important in my life.
May my mind be as clear as a lake, reflecting the face of the Divine.
May my relationship with Spirit be strong.

## AFFIRMATIONS
I am faithful to Spirit.
I am sustained by Spirit.

My boundaries support healthy relationships.
Spirit is always with me.

## ROSEWOOD *(Aniba roseodora)* WOOD

BRAZIL

### SPIRITUAL TEACHINGS

We live in a culture that values a speedy pace, somehow believing that faster is better. Every spiritual tradition counsels us against going too fast on the spiritual path. Teachers caution us to go slowly, and to integrate the teachings of each lesson before we go on to the next. They warn that becoming infused with spiritual energy too quickly, or when we are not ready, can actually cause harm. In the Hindu tradition, there are many stories of students who fasted and meditated strenuously for extended periods of time, endangering physical and mental health. In Western psychology, this is called a "spiritual emergency," and it can have the appearance of a psychotic breakdown.

Rosewood assists in spiritual development by lovingly and carefully monitoring the pace and content of the spiritual information we receive. It helps us to be in the present moment and on the present step of our path. It helps us to accept ourselves and be patient. When these qualities are in place, we naturally and effortlessly move, step by step, on our spiritual journey.

### OCCASIONS FOR USE

When we are feeling impatient about our spiritual progress.
When we are feeling blocked in our spiritual growth.
To be in the present moment of our spiritual path.

### ENERGY CENTERS

General: Brings in positive energy. Dissolves energy blockages.
Seventh: Opens us to spirituality, gently modulating the timing of the opening.

## PHYSICAL SITES
Top of head, temples, feet, hips.

## BLESSINGS
May I accept Spirit's timing as my own.
May all that I experience be in service to my spiritual growth.
May I learn to be patient.

## AFFIRMATIONS
I surrender to the wisdom of the Divine.
I patiently walk my spiritual path.
My spiritual journey is perfect.

## SANDALWOOD *(Santalum album)* WOOD

### INDIA

## SPIRITUAL TEACHINGS
Sandalwood is a profound essential oil that initiates, supports, and integrates healing on many levels. It grounds us, so we feel safe and at home on Earth. It teaches us to delight in our senses and sexuality, and to appreciate the beauty of life. It helps us to love ourselves, so that we can love others. It also helps us to maintain healthy boundaries and make good decisions about who and what we allow into our lives. Lastly, Sandalwood draws wisdom and Spirit into our being, unifying all aspects of our personality and expanding our capacity for extraordinary awareness. Sandalwood does all this, gently and calmly, so that healing unfolds naturally, like the delicate opening of a flower. Sandalwood helps us to become the embodiment of the sacred paradox of humanity—both an earthly and heavenly being, of matter and Spirit.

## OCCASIONS FOR USE
For meditation.
To improve our self-esteem.

To help us open our heart.
To help us heal relationships.

ENERGY CENTERS
General: Supports all healing. Calms and comforts.
Seventh: Encourages states of higher consciousness and a sense of unity.
Sixth: Quiets the mind. Promotes deep meditation and wisdom.
Fourth: Opens the heart to trust.
Third: Promotes positive self-esteem.
Second: Increases sexual energy.
First: Grounds and reconnects us with our sense of being.

PHYSICAL SITES
Feet, lower stomach, top and base of skull, temples, heart, middle back.

BLESSINGS
May I heal on all levels.
May I feel safe and at home on Earth.
May I accept my imperfections.

AFFIRMATIONS
I am ready to heal.
I am worthy of love.
I am of the Earth and the heavens.


SEA FENNEL *(Crythmum maritimum)* PLANT
FRANCE

SPIRITUAL TEACHINGS
Power is the ability to create, manifest, and influence our surroundings, other people, and ourselves. As we walk on our spiritual path, we grow in spiritual power. Because

we are not perfect, that power can be misused. We may incorrectly believe that our pursuits give us the right to use our power however we want, and that being "spiritual" means we can do as we please. There are many sad stories about spiritual teachers who caused great harm by stealing money, lying, or abusing students. The potential for abusing power by those "halfway up the mountain" is great.

Sea Fennel teaches about the appropriate use of power, amplifies our own power, and provides protection from being influenced by other people's inappropriate use of power. It also shows us the effects of power. If we have used it well, the results reflect the Divine. If we have misused power, such as for inappropriate personal gain, we will get immediate negative feed-back in the form of physical symptoms such as nausea or a headache, mental/emotional symptoms such as confusion, frustration, or fear, or responses from our environment such as a reprimand. The more committed we are to learning about spiritual power, the more we will receive its teachings. Those who wear the "cloak of power" lightly and invisibly can be compared to a martial arts master's gentle yet potent presence.

OCCASIONS FOR USE
When we need protection.
When we are in a power struggle with someone.
When we feel defeated or depleted by another person.
To help us learn to be a powerful yet gentle spirit.
To recover from misuse of our power.

ENERGY CENTERS
General: Helps us deal with challenging situations with strength and focus.
Third: Creates the "cloak of power." Promotes a sense of personal power and protection.

PHYSICAL SITES
Lower stomach, buttocks, solar plexus, shoulders, spine, temples.

BLESSINGS

May my power be in service to Spirit.

May I be filled with the power of Spirit.

May the cloak of power surround me, protect me, and teach me.

AFFIRMATIONS

I am powerful.

I use my power in a healthy and skillful way.

I am enveloped in the cloak of power.

## SPIKENARD *(Nardostachys jatamansi)* ROOTS
NEPAL

### SPIRITUAL TEACHINGS

To be willing to open our hearts, to truly feel and empathize with others, is an act of courage. There is an understandable tendency to cut ourselves off from feeling or responding to the terrific suffering in the world. We do this by perceiving those who suffer to be "different" from us, or by assuming that they are to blame for their predicament. However, once we make the commitment to love, how do we avoid being overwhelmed by the distress around us?

Spikenard teaches us how to be truly compassionate—feeling for others in their time of suffering—without becoming depleted. This is the blessed oil that Mary Magdalene placed on the feet of Jesus before his crucifixion. Like Mary Magdalene, we must allow compassion to touch our hearts and motivate us to pray, speak up, or act. Then, we must release our experience to Spirit. In this way, we are able to keep our hearts open to those around us, ever ready to offer compassion in times of need.

OCCASIONS FOR USE

When we feel overwhelmed by the suffering around us.

To develop compassion.

To help us understand how we can help another.

ENERGY CENTERS

General: Embodies wholeness. Promotes a sense of hope.

Seventh: Increases love and devotion for the Divine.

Fifth: Helps communication between humans and animals.

Fourth: Comforts and balances the heart, especially for people who take on the cares of the world.

PHYSICAL SITES

Temples, top of head, heart, throat, lower stomach, spine, shoulders, hands.

BLESSINGS

May I learn how to serve those who are suffering.

May the ability to love heal and strengthen me.

May I offer compassion in times of need.

AFFIRMATIONS

I am compassionate and strong.

I release this feeling of pain about the injustices in the world.

## SPRUCE  *(Picea alba* or *mariana)*  NEEDLES

CANADA

SPIRITUAL TEACHINGS

Spruce teaches us to walk our spiritual path with "practical feet," moving forward and making choices with grounded wisdom and intuitive understanding. Spruce supports intuition and also teaches us about compassion, for ourselves as well as others. It allows us to feel compassion despite our mistakes and fears. It also helps us to accept and communicate information we receive intuitively about other people in a caring way. Spruce opens the mind and heart while clearing away negativity and outmoded thoughts. This helps us to see and speak truthfully, and to feel and act with compassionate wisdom.

OCCASIONS FOR USE
To act on our intuition.
To communicate our intuitive understanding with skill and compassion.
When negative thoughts, feelings, and judgements are blocking our intuition.

ENERGY CENTERS
Sixth: Develops intuition.
Fifth: Assists in compassionate communication.
Fourth: Develops compassion.
First: Grounds.

PHYSICAL SITES
Center of forehead, temples, heart, throat, feet, knees, lower stomach.

BLESSINGS
May I open my mind and heart to the truth of Spirit.
May my mind and heart be compassionate.
Bless my words so that they may be a blessing to others.

AFFIRMATIONS
I walk my spiritual path with practical feet.
My wisdom is embodied in my daily life and practice.
I communicate my intuitive understandings with wisdom and compassion.
I release negative energy.

## VETIVER *(Vetiveria zizanoides)* ROOTS
### INDONESIA

### SPIRITUAL TEACHINGS
Vetiver profoundly balances and grounds us so that we are receptive to spiritual energy. It reminds us that our task as humans is to embody Spirit and reflect the wisdom that is gained from uniting matter and Spirit. We do not have to choose between heaven and Earth—the Divine is always here and now. This allows us to feel safe and calm, along with a deep sense of belonging that is our birthright.

### OCCASIONS FOR USE
When we are feeling ungrounded or confused.

When we feel unsafe in the world.

When our personal boundaries are vulnerable and weak.

When we are feeling exhausted, depleted, or disconnected from our spiritual path.

### ENERGY CENTERS
General: Clears and cleanses a room. Brings in positive energy. Protects the energy field. Grounds and centers. Protects against over-sensitivity.

Seventh: Promotes spiritual calmness.

Sixth: Promotes wisdom.

Third: Promotes positive self-esteem.

First: Calms and grounds. Promotes strength and a deep sense of belonging.

### PHYSICAL SITES
Feet, lower stomach, temples, heart, full back, joints.

### BLESSINGS
May I be grounded and protected.

May I be filled with grace.

May I be wise in the choices I make.

AFFIRMATIONS

I am safe and protected.

I am grounded.

I am open to Spirit.

Spirit fills and grounds me.

## YLANG YLANG *(Cananga odorata)* BLOSSOMS
MADAGASCAR

SPIRITUAL TEACHINGS

Fear is a part of our emotional repertoire. It can be an important companion—alerting us to the presence of real danger and making us acutely aware so we can protect ourselves. However, fear has a negative side. It can paralyze our personal growth when it is a reaction to change and transformation. Fear can distort our awareness of the present and the potential it holds for the unfolding of a promising future. Immobilizing, reactive fear cannot distinguish between the threat of death and the helpful death of old patterns that occur with each step forward on our spiritual path. Ylang Ylang helps us to confidently deal with our fears and to recognize whether or not they are appropriate or useful. It also helps us to be courageous and at peace.

OCCASIONS FOR USE

When we are feeling fearful.

When we are preparing for, or in the process of, making changes in our life.

When we want to feel confident and assured.

ENERGY CENTERS

General: Promotes feelings of peace. Dispels anger and fear.

Third: Promotes self-confidence and enthusiasm.

Second: Increases sexuality. Helps to unite emotional and sexual natures.

## PHYSICAL SITES

Kidneys, temples, lower stomach, ankles, knees, joints, hips.

## BLESSINGS

May I release fears, old or new, that prevent me from moving forward.
May I understand the lessons of fear.
Bless me during this time of change.

## AFFIRMATIONS

I am a person of courage.
I embrace change.
I release fear.

CHAPTER THREE
# CREATING A SACRED SPACE FOR AROMATHERAPY ANOINTING

"*S*acred space" refers to a time and a place that is designated for and devoted to experiencing a connection to the Divine. It provides the setting and environment for anointing and can be created any time and any place by *clearing the area, protecting the area, asking for guidance, and setting intention.* These steps can be accomplished in a matter of moments, or they can be a part of a planned, lengthy ceremony. Sacred space is enhanced by the addition of affirmations, candles, colors, crystals, the elements, essential oils, flower essences, food, drink, images, incense, prayers, sound, stones, and visualizations. Many spiritual traditions remind us that all space and all time is sacred. "Creating sacred space" simply helps us to become particularly aware of the spiritual dimension within and around us.

## CLEARING THE AREA

Just as we clear a space on the kitchen counter when we prepare food, so too must we clear an area energetically when we want a place for our sacred work such as anointing. This is a conscious, three-step process: 1) First, initiate a shift in your consciousness, focusing body, mind, and spirit on the Divine. 2) Release all other thoughts and intentions. 3) Dedicate the area to the Divine. You can include specific helpful techniques such as taking a deep breath and releasing it, with the purpose of making a transition into sacred awareness, or using essential oils in a diffuser or mist to cleanse the area and support a sense of spirituality. Oils especially appropriate for this purpose are Juniper, Lavender, Cedarwood, and Eucalyptus. Another technique is saying an affirmation such as, "The area is now clear and ready for the anointing." Note: To make a mist, mix ten to fifteen drops of essential oil in four ounces of water in a misting bottle. Shake before each use.

## PROTECTING THE AREA

"Protecting the area" refers to creating a safe, comfortable, secure, and contained space in which to give or receive an anointing. A contained space has a type of semi-permeable, energetic membrane in which all that supports the sacredness of the space can enter, and all that would interfere is kept out. This is accomplished by physical actions such as turning off the phone, putting out a "do not disturb" sign, or drawing a boundary such as a circle or square, as well as energetically by visualizing a wall of white light around the area. Essential oils that protect sacred space include Rosemary, Vetiver, Rose, Angelica, Bay Laurel, Geranium, and Pine. They can be diffused or misted in the space, or used to anoint objects in the area to establish the protective boundary.

## ASKING FOR GUIDANCE

"Asking for guidance" invites any special spiritual being or guide to be present during an anointing, such as Jesus, Buddha, Quan Yin, a particular angel, or an animal. It can also be someone you love who has died, such as your grandmother or a teacher. Invite one or more guides, as long as they are meaningful to you. There is a saying in the Christian tradition, "Ask and you shall receive." The technique of asking for guidance is as simple as this. Direct your sincere invitation and request to those you want present, and they will be there.

A guide is invited for support and to protect you from negative influences. Their presence amplifies both your intention and the potency of the anointing oil, and attempts to ensure that what you ask for will be for the highest good—for you and for all. The invitation to be present also provides an opportunity to ask for a guide's blessing. At any time during an anointing ceremony, feel free to ask the guide(s) to be with you and help you.

## SETTING INTENTION

"Setting intention" is declaring, silently or out loud, the purpose for which you are anointing, such as, "This anointing is to support me as I begin my new job." (See Chapter 5 for a wide variety of occasions for anointing.) Affirmations such as "I am strong and confident during this time of change and opportunity" are appropriate, and blessings such as "May this new job be rewarding and satisfying" can also be used. A single word that represents a desired state can set intention, such as "peace" or "joy." Lastly, intention can be set by a visualization of a desired state such as an image of a calm lake, or a rose opening to its full bloom.

## ENHANCING SACRED SPACE

Following are several ways to enhance sacred space. These techniques amplify and focus intention and can be incorporated into any or all of the four steps involved in creating sacred space: clearing the area, protecting the area, asking for guidance, and setting intention. Though they are not essential for anointing, many people find them especially meaningful as well as enjoyable.

### AFFIRMATIONS

Affirmations are positive statements that focus consciousness and intent. They are said with sincerity, one or several times, silently or out loud. One method we find effective is to say the affirmation three times silently, then three times out loud. Imagine sending the affirmation into the base of the skull to become a part of your belief system, both conscious and unconscious. The mind has enormous capacity to impact reality, and affirmations activate that power.

In her ground-breaking book, *I Deserve Love*, Sondra Ray writes about affirmations and how to work with them to identify and change old belief systems, along with the emotional/thought patterns that sustain them. She suggests several guidelines for creating affirmations, which other writers and practitioners have added to and refined.

* Keep the affirmation brief and clear.
* Work on one thing at a time.
* Avoid the word "try."
* Speak in the present tense such as "I am healing now," or "Each day I am more and more healthy," instead of "I will be getting healthier," or "I am going to be healthier."
* Keep the language positive such as "I feel strong and confident," instead of "I don't feel uncomfortable."
* Make affirmations believable such as "I am uniquely beautiful," instead of "I am the most beautiful person in the world." Or "I deserve abundance and I call wealth into my life now," instead of "Next week I am going to have a million dollars."

If you have trouble believing your affirmation, try this exercise using an affirmation journal.

* Write the affirmation on the left side of the page.
* On the right-hand side, write your first response. For example, Affirmation: "I am confident." Response: "Oh yeah? I don't know what I am doing."
* Do this ten times, and notice that what is written on the right side are your underlying negative beliefs, thoughts, and feelings that are preventing you from believing your affirmation.
* As you work with this, two things may happen. One, the negative responses begin to change as you become conscious of them. Two, you can create new affirmations in response to the negativity. They may be general, such as "I am willing to release my negative thoughts," or specific, such as "I release all outmoded thoughts that prevent me from being confident."

## BLESSINGS / PRAYERS

Blessings and prayers are requests or calls to Spirit to help fulfill personal intention, such as those for support, transformation, or healing. Ask that Spirit grace you with what you feel you need, and what your heart desires. We often include the caveat "If it is thy will." The source of wisdom in blessings and prayers is Spirit, rather than one-self. Blessings and prayers are very helpful to use when creating sacred space for anointing. Two of our favorites are "May this space be filled with Spirit" and "Bless this time and this place."

## CANDLES

In many spiritual traditions, light symbolizes how the Divine illuminates the human condition. Lighting a candle and saying a blessing or affirmation is a simple way to bring light, warmth, and awareness to our purpose of anointing.

Choosing a particular shape or color for the candle aligns it with various intentions and amplifies the power and focus of the flickering light. Round candles are symbolic of the Earth and female energy, square represents building and creating, and a taper signifies Spirit. The meanings of the colors of your candles are described below.

## COLORS

Color is all around us—an integral part of daily life. We are affected by the unique energetic patterns of different colors as they travel through our eyes and influence our brain. Generally, the cooler colors of blue, indigo, and violet relax us, and the warmer color of red, orange, and yellow energize us.

Color is used in sacred space in many forms—some favorites are flowers, beads, candles, and cloth. The following is a traditional interpretation of color.

RED Enthusiasm, passion, celebration, inspiration, courage, sexuality, leadership.
ORANGE Enthusiasm, health, happiness, joy, optimism.
YELLOW Knowledge, mental clarity, curiosity, cheerfulness, objectivity.
GREEN Healing, harmony, prosperity, security, stability, cleanliness, balance.
BLUE Introspection, calmness, coolness, concentration.
INDIGO Introspection, calmness, devotion, logical thought, present awareness.
VIOLET Independence, royalty, spiritual vitality, peace, creativity.

We have experienced additional impressions of using color in sacred space:

PINK OR ROSE Love, compassion.

WHITE Spirituality, purity, inner silence.

GOLD Spirituality, abundance.

LAVENDER To release negativity.

TURQUOISE Detached compassion, Christ consciousness.

INDIGO Compassionate mind, Buddha consciousness.

SILVER Spiritual protection, spiritual evolution.

## CRYSTALS

Crystals are minerals from the Earth that hold, receive, transmit, and amplify energy. Both science and industry use them in computers and electronic components because of this energetic capacity. In healing and spiritual work, the capacity of crystals to focus and increase intention makes them an invaluable addition for enhancing sacred space and aromatherapy anointing.

Although there is a great deal of information available about the various crystals and what they do, we encourage you to use your preference and intuition in choosing one for your sacred space. You may choose a crystal because of its color (blue for relaxation), texture (smooth to help things go smoothly in your life), shape (straight with a pointed end to help you move along your life's path), or simply because you feel drawn to it.

Because crystals hold energy, they should be *cleared* and then *programmed* before each use. Most crystal books will teach you how to do this, but we recommend swabbing the crystal with Cedarwood oil, then putting it in a bowl of salt water, preferably in the sun, for a few hours to clear it. You can use actual ocean water to do this, or mix one teaspoon of sea salt in one cup of spring water. The crystal can then be programmed in a variety of ways. We use affirmations, blessings, and anointing with a drop of essential oil. To bring balance and harmony, we say, "May this crystal balance the body, mind, heart, and spirit of whoever it touches," while we anoint the crystal with Lavender. For grounding, we may say while touching obsidian with a drop of Vetiver, "May this obsidian ground this room and all who come into it, and provide safety and security."

The following chart provides information about many different crystals. You may want to include one or more of them when you create sacred space for aromatherapy anointing.

| NAME | COLOR | CHARACTERISTICS |
| --- | --- | --- |
| Amethyst | Lavender | Balances, promotes peace, supports intuition. |
| Black onyx | Black | Grounds, promotes stamina, supports self-control. |
| Citrine | Yellow/gold | Promotes clarity, confidence, success, abundance. |
| Flourite | Purple | Represents spiritual truth, supports intuition. |
| Flourite | Clear | Represents serenity. |
| Flourite | Blue | Provides emotional protection. |
| Flourite | Green | Supports healing on all levels. |
| Jasper | Red | Provides physical protection, supports emotional healing, balances, nurtures. |
| Jasper | Yellow | Strengthens personal will, supports emotional healing, balances. |
| Moldavite | Dark green | Supports spirit journeys, promotes higher states of consciousness. |
| Obsidian | Black | Grounds, stabilizes. |
| Peridot | Olive or yellow-green | Supports the healing of relationships, replenishes the heart center. |
| Quartz | Clear | Supports healing, clears the body/mind, strengthens. |
| Rose quartz | Pink/rose | Supports the healing of the heart center, comforts, opens the heart and mind to love. |
| Sugilite | Purple | Helps to develop healing abilities, spirituality, and intuition. |

| NAME | COLOR | CHARACTERISTICS |
|------|-------|-----------------|
| Tanzanite | Purple/blue | Helps to connect us with spirit guides. |
| Tiger's Eye | Red | Helps to release fear and anxiety, promotes security. |
| Tiger's Eye | Gold | Supports personal will power. |
| Tiger's Eye | Blue | Assists communication. |
| Topaz | Golden | Promotes self-confidence and abundance. |
| Topaz | Blue | Supports psychic vision. |
| Topaz | Pink | Supports the giving and receiving of love. |
| Topaz | White | Supports spirituality. |
| Tourmaline | Red | Energizes. Tourmaline Pink Helps to open the heart center. |
| Tourmaline | Green | Supports healing. |
| Tourmaline | Watermelon | Helps to heal a wounded heart center. |
| Tourmaline | Pink | Helps to open heart center. |

## ELEMENTS

"Elements" refers to substances that make up the material world. Different cultures and traditions have different systems that represent the elements. Chinese medicine speaks of the five elements of water, wood, fire, earth, and metal. The African Dagara tradition, mentioned in the earlier interview with Jan Boddie and Marystella Church in Chapter 1, also has five elements but they are different ones: fire, water, earth, nature, and mineral. We use a four-element system: earth, water, fire, and air. This is commonly used by Native American people such as the Cherokee and the Lakota Sioux.

Each element has a physical, emotional, and spiritual aspect. Including them in your sacred space is a way to connect to Mother Earth. You may incorporate all of them for a sense of balance and completeness, or you can focus on one to bring that specific quality into your life.

### WATER

The water element represents the fluid realm of emotion, empathy, connection, and deep understanding. It can help bring movement into any area of your life that feels stagnant. The element of water can be present in the anointing area by including a bowl of water, a picture of water such as a lake or waterfall, a shell, or a pearl. It is portrayed by the colors blue or green.

## EARTH

The earth element grounds and assists us in manifesting goals in a concrete way. It also relates to our life's work, helping us to consistently commit to and pursue our goals. Earth helps us to feel and be at home in our physical body. Include earth when creating sacred space to support your personal path. The element of earth can be represented by an earthenware bowl, a stone, earth (dirt) in a container, a crystal, or a picture. It is symbolized by the colors of brown, black, dark red, and dark orange.

## FIRE

The fire element inspires, energizes, cleanses, and supports intuition and visualization. The cleansing nature of fire helps us to express our true self. Use fire for energy and inspiration, and to release outmoded habits. Fire can be represented in your sacred space by lighting a candle, burning incense, turning on an electric light, or displaying a picture of fire. The element of fire is represented by the colors red, orange, and yellow.

## AIR

The element of air relates to the mind, thoughts, and communication. It is used to promote mental clarity and focus in order to better understand and communicate thoughts more effectively. It can be used whenever you need to think carefully about a particular situation, understand an event in your life, or communicate well. You can also use it to identify and release negative thoughts. The air element can be represented in your sacred space by a feather, a fan, a statue of a bird, a picture of the sky, and the sound of bells or flutes. Its color is a very pale blue.

*Note: Depending on your intention of sacred space, you may want to combine elements such as mud for water and earth, or blowing on a burning herb for fire and air.*

## ESSENTIAL OILS (AROMATHERAPY)

Essential oils are used to enhance sacred space in a variety of ways. They can be diffused or misted in a room to impart their particular energy, purpose, and blessing as well as their fragrance. They can also simply be placed in the area in their bottle, or a few drops put in a bowl. Find an oil that supports your intention and whose fragrance pleases you.

Some common essential oils diffused to clear and cleanse the area are Cedarwood, Elemi, Eucalyptus, Juniper, Lavender, Pine, Rosemary, and Vetiver. To set intention and fill the space with positive energy use Bergamot, Cedarwood, Lavender, Lemon, Orange, Neroli, Rose, Rosewood, or Vetiver. For protection use Fennel, Rosemary, Juniper, or Vetiver.

## FLOWER ESSENCES

Flower essences are liquid preparations made from a wide variety of flowers; they contain the flowers' energetic patterns or ethereal imprints. They are used as a catalyst for the transformation of emotions, attitudes, and patterns of behavior, and they encourage the awakening of our innate ability to be whole and well in body, mind, and spirit.

Flower essences influence the subtle realm—energy centers and subtle bodies—and provide support for your intentions. When creating sacred space, they can be taken internally, applied topically, used in a mister, set in the area in their bottle, or put in a bowl of water. We frequently use flower essences in creating sacred space. Some of our favorites include:

WILD OAT to help discover our life purpose.

HORN OF PLENTY to dedicate the space to universal love.

AGRIMONY to help communicate our true feelings.

SELF HEAL to help in a healing process.

IRIS to encourage creativity.

ASPEN for inner confidence and feeling secure.

CERATO to help us trust in our own inner wisdom.

HOLLY to open our heart and unite us with Divine love.

MIMULUS to help us overcome our fears.

OAK to help us take care of ourselves when we are depleted.

STAR OF BETHLEHEM to help us recover from physical or emotional shock.

WHITE CHESTNUT to help us let go of worries and unhappy memories.

WILLOW to help us be optimistic and have faith.

## FOOD OR DRINK

Food or drink placed in sacred space represents how Spirit nourishes us. The food can be something special—a delicacy that reminds us of the precious nature of the sacred—or it can be something ordinary to remind us that the sacred is always with us. The food can be eaten by the participants after the ceremony, or disposed of in a special manner. For example, bread may be placed in the area to represent deep, life-giving sustenance, and then shared later. A glass of wine or juice can represent the sweetness and life force of the Holy, and after the anointing, it can be poured on the ground as an offering and blessing to the Earth.

## IMAGES

Many spiritual traditions use images to help followers remember and focus on the Holy. Representations, statues, and pictures are used in sacred spaces such as churches, temples, and meditation rooms. Especially familiar are those of blessed beings, such as Buddha, Jesus, Mary, and Quan Yin. Yet a sacred image can be anything that is dear to you and represents the sacred—a picture of a holy place, a tile painted with a sacred geometric design, a carving of an animal, a bowl painted with stars, a crystal, or a special stone. Used in a setting for anointing, the image you choose should expand and bring clarity to your spiritual vision.

## INCENSE / SMUDGING

Incense is traditionally a combination of plant gums, resins, and aromatic herbs that release their fragrances when burned. You can find incense in its natural form or shaped into sticks and cones in a variety of fragrances—from sweet to resinous. Many of the very sweet incenses from India are intended to invite a Divine presence. Lavender incense clears, cleanses, and balances. Pine helps to remove emotional or energetic obstacles and also refreshes the air.

For your sacred space, the fragrance of incense can be used to fill the area with your intention, or you can place the unburned incense in the area with the intention that its simple presence assist you in your purpose. (This is preferable if there are people present who are bothered by the smoke that incense creates.)

Smudging is similar to burning incense, but instead of resin, loose leaves or bound herbs are lit with a flame, blown out, and then allowed to smolder, releasing both fragrance and smoke. The herbs usually need to be fanned in order to keep them smoldering, so we use a feather to wave back and forth over the smudge, which sends the scent throughout the room. Common smudges include sage to clear and cleanse a room, and sweetgrass to fill the area with positive energy. *Always remember that after you clear a space, you need to fill it with your desired intention.*

## SOUNDS

The energy and vibration of sound can fill and change the feeling of an area, as well as alter consciousness. The gradual dissipation of sound as it fades into silence helps to clear, focus, and center your mind, promoting a sense of sacred space. Bells, rattles, and chimes are used to disperse negative energy. Music, appropriately chosen, amplifies intention. Your voice can be used as an instrument to bless and heal by toning, chanting, or singing. Specific word sounds are used in different traditions to designate sacred space, such as the "Ho" of Native Americans and the "Amen" of Christians.

When preparing sacred space, a bell can be sounded to clear and protect the area. A favorite song or chant might come before, during, or after the anointing. Blessings and affirmations can be sung as a way to align with Divine will. During more formal ceremonies such as weddings or birthdays, music that is special to the participants may be played to set the tone for the occasion.

STONES

Many indigenous peoples, such as Native Americans and the Aborigines of Australia, considered stones to be ancient, wise beings, filled with a consciousness of history and the rhythm of life. Their language reflects their belief in the animate nature of stones, referring to them, roughly translated, as "the stone people." Stones represent ancient wisdom, the cycle of nature, and the strength of the Earth. If you would like these qualities present during an anointing, place stones in the area.

In choosing a stone, you may be drawn to its color, texture, or form. It can put you in touch, through it unique qualities, with something you desire. A green rock may represent abundance and healing. A stone smoothed by water may remind you of the ways in which the difficulties of life can shape, smooth, and even beautify the soul. Ruah keeps a rock in her healing room that is formed in the shape of a wise old woman. Before working with clients, she anoints it with Vetiver to help connect with Earth and grounded wisdom.

TENDING TO THE SENSES

The five physical senses—seeing, touching, tasting, hearing, and smelling—are avenues of communication to the psyche. When their input is positive and pleasant, they provide nourishment for the soul. For the anointing, you may tend to all the senses as a part of your way to enhance sacred space, or choose those that are particularly meaningful to you.

VISION Objects of beauty, flowers, favorite colors, or pictures of special places.

TOUCH / FEELING Comfortable places to sit, touching or holding a special object, feeling the texture of a special garment such as a meditation scarf.

HEARING Soothing music, moving water, a bell, a song, a chant, or a particular word such as "Om."

SMELL Incense, essential oils, fresh flowers, or dried herbs.

TASTE A special food or drink consumed before or after an anointing, an offering to Spirit, a symbol of the way in which the sacred nourishes us.

VISUALIZATIONS

Visualization, or imagery, is an affirmation in the form of a mental picture. To visualize, create an image in your mind of what you want, and imbue that image with your intention. The image can be a literal representation or symbolic. For example, if you want physical healing, imagine that the body is healthy and whole. See it, feel it, and imagine it as reality. A symbolic image for health and healing might be a beautiful opened flower, a strong animal, or even a car—new, well-kept, and running perfectly. A visualization can be static such as the image of an opened flower, or moving such as a flower in the process of opening.

When you use visualization, be sure to affirm what the image represents: "Every time I imagine this flower opening, my immune system becomes even stronger." After affirming your intention once or twice, the image itself will trigger the intention without you having to state it, although you can continue to do so.

Visualizations are well suited for clearing an area and setting intention when creating sacred space. To clear an area, imagine a white, gold, or silver light spinning from your hands as you "sweep" the room, or the breath of spirit blowing out all negativity. To set intention, simply align your visualization with the purpose of the anointing. For example, if your intention is to be balanced, imagine a color that represents balance, such as lavender, or visualize a symbol of balance such as a scale or a body walking on balanced feet. Allow yourself to create and discover what works well for you—whatever is "right" for you will be "right" for the anointing.

CLOSING SACRED SPACE

When sacred space is created for anointing, it must also be "closed" after the work is finished to signify a completion and a return to ordinary consciousness. In essence, it is undoing what was originally done to create the sacred space. It may mean blowing out the candles, pouring out the bowl of water, or snuffing out the incense. You can use a phrase or word such as "Blessed be" or "Amen," or a closing intention statement such as "I release all that has been said, done, and experienced here to Spirit."

Affirmations can also be used such as "I close this space now and intend that all that has happened here be for the benefit of all beings." Finally, thank Spirit and hold gratitude in your heart. Afterwards, give yourself and your participants a few moments to transition fully out of that sacred time and place.

## CREATING A SPECIAL PLACE FOR YOUR AROMATHERAPY ANOINTING OILS

You may want to create a small area of sacred space in your home or office to keep your anointing oils. Some people refer to this as a personal altar—an ever-present, daily reminder of the sacred. You may have already done this, in some fashion, without realizing it. Include any of the elements mentioned in this chapter, as well as personal mementos, such as pictures of family and friends. Remember, however, to take care of it—keep it clean, and remove items if they lose meaning for you.

## CHAPTER FOUR

# THE ANOINTING TOUCH

*A*romatherapy anointing is a gentle, intentional touch to the body using essential oils diluted in vegetable oil. This quintessential contact directs a spiritual blessing to the human, physical form. Its impact is directly related to your intention, your hands, and the nature of touch—the most significant elements of this ancient, sacred technique.

Intention is the deep, inner embrace of a spiritual objective and purpose that shifts reality on a subtle level to align with the Divine. Intention is also being clear about the purpose of the anointing. This potent state of mind affects both the one being anointed as well as the one anointing.

Your hands, symbols of giving and receiving, are the perfect instruments to administer an anointing. They are wondrous in their ability to help—yourself as well as another person. All of who you are, and what you intend, can be expressed through your hands. In the case of anointing, they are the tools of the messenger—the means by which a sacred gift is delivered.

Touch is a powerful way to connect and communicate with another human being. It is a universal language and fulfills a basic human need—to touch and be touched. It has immense impact on the psyche and is of monumental importance to physical, psychological, and spiritual well-being. In *Touching: The Human Significance of Skin*, Ashley Montagu says, "Where touching begins, there love and humanity also begin...."

Touching the body with anointing oil anchors and amplifies the intention of the anointing on a physical level, helping to attract what is needed as well as to embody it. It also deepens and strengthens a sense of purpose and connection to the Divine. Rudolph Steiner, the founder of Anthroposophy, believed that human beings could not become conscious of the Divine without touch—a particularly meaningful concept in respect to anointing.

To anoint another person or yourself, put a drop or two of an aromatherapy anointing oil on the index or middle fingertip of your right hand if right-handed, and left hand if left-handed. Then use one of the following methods, accompanied by a blessing or affirmation. (Where to place the anointing oil is discussed below.)

* Simply touch the area, then say the blessing or affirmation.
* Touch the area for the length of time it takes to say the blessing or affirmation.
* Touch with a clockwise motion to send the blessing or affirmation inward.
* Touch with a counter-clockwise motion to assist in the letting go or releasing of what is no longer needed.
* Touch with a downward stroke to symbolize bringing Spirit into the body.
* Touch with the motion of a cross. The vertical stroke symbolizes inviting Spirit into the body. The horizontal stroke aligns Spirit with the Earth. This is also the traditional symbol of the Christian faith, representing Christ consciousness.
* Touch with the motion of a five-pointed star. This signifies protection and a connection with nature. It also aligns the body, mind, and spirit with the highest of human potential.
* Touch with the motion of a circle, clockwise, to invoke healing on all levels, to honor the sacredness of Earth and the body, and to invite a sense of completion.
* Touch with the motion of the symbol of an energy center to attract the qualities of that particular center. (See illustrations below.)
* Touch with the motion of any symbol that is especially meaningful to you or the person being anointed.

There are three approaches for deciding where on the body to anoint: body symbology, subtle anatomy, and physical symptoms. You may relate to one of these more than another, or you may be comfortable using all three systems individually or combined. Any are acceptable, as long as you and the person being anointed find them relevant.

For those people or situations when touching the body is not appropriate or comfortable, an anointing can be given off the body. Simply hold your finger with intention several inches away from the area of the body to be anointed, and bless or affirm as desired.

## BODY SYMBOLOGY

Body symbology identifies various parts of the physical body with symbolic meanings. For example, on a tangible level, the heart is an organ that pumps blood to circulate through the body. On a symbolic level, it is associated with giving and receiving love, as well as the harbor for grief and joy.

Following is a list of symbolic associations that are useful for aromatherapy anointing. It is the result of tradition, research, and personal experience. It is not definitive, and we encourage you to be open to your own experiences, whether cognitive or intuitive. Anoint where you are drawn to anoint, using this list as a general guideline. Working with essential oils in the subtle realm tends to increase intuition and body awareness, so don't be surprised if you discover symbolic associations of your own.

TOP OF HEAD To invite Divine guidance.

BASE OF SKULL To access instinctual abilities, wisdom, and memories. To strengthen intentions. To promote a sense of well-being.

CENTER OF FOREHEAD To increase intuition and knowing.

SPINE To help give and receive support. To have the ability "to carry on."

SHOULDERS To support carrying life's experiences, lessons, and challenges with joy, pride, and ease.

BACK Full length: To balance the body and emotions. Lower back: To create financial ease. Middle back: To release feelings of guilt. Upper back, between shoulder blades, behind heart: To receive and give love.

SENSES To open hearing, seeing, smelling, and tasting to higher knowing and expanded perception. Ears: To hear the truth and to promote receptivity to inner and outer information. Eyes: To "see" or perceive more clearly. Mouth: To "taste" or experience life more fully. Nose: To "sniff out" or distinguish reality. Note: *Anoint around, but not in, the ears, eyes, nose, or mouth.* You can also anoint above the body near these areas, without touching.

TEMPLES To support moments of prayer or meditation. To relieve worry and promote mental clarity.

JAW OR THROAT To provide support for speaking the truth.

BREASTS To give and receive mothering or nurturing support. To be nourished by feminine energy.

HEART To invite in and send out love. To expand the capacity to love. To be able to feel and accept love. To promote a sense of peace.

HANDS To bless whatever is touched. To bring the experience of meaning to all one does. To promote creative expression.

PALMS OF THE HANDS To support receiving abundance and experiencing prosperity. To activate healing energy in the hands.

SOLAR PLEXUS To support trusting and understanding instincts or "gut" reactions.

STOMACH, LOWER To attract what is desired. To protect from negative influences. To help "digest" and integrate experiences, feelings, and information.

HIPS To provide support for moving forward in life.

BUTTOCKS To be in touch with the "seat of power."

KNEE To support emotional flexibility, and responsible and responsive action. To help release emotions.

ANKLE To be able to receive pleasure.

FEET To walk a spiritual or life path with intention. To ground and balance. To feel connected to the Earth and its wisdom. To move forward in life.

PULSE POINTS (BEHIND EAR, INNER WRIST, ANKLE, INNER ELBOW, BEHIND KNEE)
To bless and strengthen the life force throughout the body. To connect with vitality and joy.

JOINTS  To support an easy response to changes in life's direction.

LEFT SIDE OF THE BODY  For issues about a mother, the past, or the feminine.

RIGHT SIDE OF THE BODY  For issues about a father, the future, or the masculine.

LIVER  For issues about anger.

KIDNEYS  For issues about fear.

LUNGS  For issues about grief.

SHOULDER BLADES  For paternal support. To connect with the Divine father.

AN EXAMPLE OF USING BODY SYMBOLOGY WITH
AROMATHERAPY ANOINTING OILS

A group of women friends decided to create a ceremony to help them face their fears about money. Their intention was to increase their sense of deserving prosperity as well as competency about finances. They created a prosperity anointing blend with Ginger for gratitude and abundance, and Bay Laurel to change their attitude about money. They bought a beautiful statue together of Lakshmi, the Hindu goddess of abundance.

Each woman anointed herself:

* On the temples saying, "I release all my old thoughts about money and invite an attitude of abundance."
* On both palms saying, "I deserve prosperity."
* On the solar plexus saying, "I am prosperous."
* Over the heart saying, "I love prosperity and am grateful for all the abundance in my life."
* On the forehead saying, "I have a new attitude about money. It is easy for me to understand finances. Money flows easily to me now."

Then, as a group, they anointed the statue in the same areas.

## SUBTLE ANATOMY

The subtle anatomy of the body is comprised of energy centers and subtle bodies. There are seven primary energy centers, also known as chakras, located along the spine from the tailbone to the top of the head. They receive, assimilate, and transmit various forms of energy, playing a vital role in our state of consciousness and emotional nature. The subtle bodies are levels of energy that pass through the physical body outward from the skin. We identify these levels as etheric (closest to the body), astral, mental, and spiritual (furthest from the body). Together they form an energetic structure that is referred to as the aura, auric field, electromagnetic field, biofield, and energy field.

For the purpose of anointing, understanding the energy centers provides a way to direct our intention and interpret the many aspects of our lives, such as our sense of security, relationship with others, self-image, ability to love and feel compassion, communication skills, intelligence, intuition, and connection to the Divine. Understanding the energy centers also helps us work effectively with essential oils, because essential oils have physical, mental, emotional, and spiritual properties that resonate with corresponding attributes of the energy centers.

Each one of these centers has a particular location along the spine, is connected to the physical functioning of specific organs and glands, and is associated with certain psychological issues. Following is a brief description of these attributes, the qualities that can be accessed for anointing, and the energy centers' spiritual teachings.

### FIRST CENTER

Base Center. Located at the base of the spine. Associated with the intestines and adrenal glands. Concerned with self-preservation and survival. Anoint to invite a strong connection with Mother Earth, to ground, stabilize, feel secure, feel safe, connect with abundance, and to feel "at home" in the body and on the Earth. Teaches us about the embodiment of Spirit, and the sacredness of the physical world.

## SECOND CENTER

Sacral Center. Located two inches below the navel. Associated with the reproductive organs and glands. Concerned with sexuality, creativity, and relationships. Anoint to allow feelings to flow, to access enthusiasm, sensuality, creativity, pleasure, and to encourage or improve relationships. Teaches us about aligning sexuality, emotions, and feelings with Spirit.

## THIRD CENTER

Solar Plexus Center. Located two inches above the navel. Associated with the digestive system, liver, and pancreas. Concerned with personal power and will, self-worth, social identity, and likes and dislikes. Anoint to build confidence, self-acceptance, and self-esteem, to assist in achieving goals, to develop personal will and integrity, and to attract what is wanted in life. Teaches us about the personality developing to be of service to the Divine.

## FOURTH CENTER

Heart Center. Located in the center of the chest. Associated with the heart, lungs, and thymus gland. Concerned with love, compassion, and the connection to friends and family. Anoint to accept and nurture oneself and others, to love, to connect with community, to discover life's purpose, and to feel and express compassion, joy, and peace. Teaches us about the connection with the infinite, abundant love that is Spirit.

## FIFTH CENTER

Throat Center. Located in the center of the throat. Associated with the neck, throat, and thyroid gland. Concerned with communication (both speaking and listening). Anoint to express the truth freely, safely, completely, and appropriately, to be comfortable with silence and able to listen to others as well as one's inner voice, to manage time well, and to connect with Divine will. Teaches us about the personal will aligning with the Divine will to become an instrument of the sacred.

SIXTH CENTER

Third Eye or Brow Center. Located on the forehead, just above and between the eyes. Associated with the eyes, pituitary, and the hypothalamus. Concerned with intellect, understanding, intuition, and dreams. Anoint to develop and balance the intuitive and rational minds, to assist in memory and psychic development, and to increase self-awareness and self-knowledge. Teaches us about the healing, balancing, and expanding of the human mind so it can be touched by the mind of Spirit.

SEVENTH CENTER

Crown Center. Located on the top of the head. Associated with the brain, the central nervous system, and the pineal gland. Concerned with spirituality, faith, and higher states of consciousness. Anoint to promote enlightenment, to deepen faith, to achieve higher states of consciousness, and to connect with the Divine. Teaches us about surrendering to the mystery of the Divine, becoming one with Spirit.

Symbols of the energy centers can be used in aromatherapy anointing by holding their image in your mind as you anoint, or by actually drawing them with the oil. The following are suggested symbols for each energy center.

*Note: The symbols associated with the energy centers vary amongst different schools of thought. Symbols are created and used because they communicate without words, representing an idea or group of ideas. For example, we portray the base energy center as a square, giving the sense of solidity and stability—both qualities of this center. Due to individual interpretation, there is a variety of associated symbols. Feel free to use any symbol that is meaningful to you and gives you a sense of that particular center. You may also create your own.*

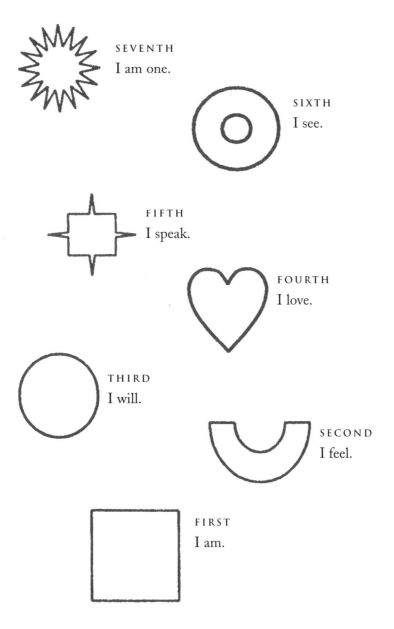

SEVENTH
I am one.

SIXTH
I see.

FIFTH
I speak.

FOURTH
I love.

THIRD
I will.

SECOND
I feel.

FIRST
I am.

## AN EXAMPLE OF USING THE ENERGY CENTERS WITH AROMATHERAPY ANOINTING OILS

A couple was having difficulty in conceiving a child. Together they created an anointing blend to provide emotional support during the difficult medical procedures. It contained Frangipani for the fertility of Mother Earth, Jasmine to honor the blend of the Divine masculine and feminine, Rose for love, and a touch of Orange for great joy. Each night they would lovingly anoint each other's energy centers:

* The Second for opening to creative, fertile sexuality.
* The Third for invoking the capacity to manifest what is desired into reality.
* The Fourth for honoring the love between them.
* The Fifth for aligning with Divine will and inviting the child that was waiting for them.

Then they said a blessing or affirmation that came from the heart—something new each time.

They reported later, after having a daughter, that they believed that the mutual anointing not only helped them to conceive, but also brought them much closer to each other in a very intimate and spiritual way.

## PHYSICAL SYMPTOMS

The third approach to anointing the body is in relationship with physical symptoms. Touching parts of the body that are wounded or symptomatic of illness is a natural human response, worldwide. Aromatherapy anointing is a wonderful way to accompany this innate instinct.

To anoint a symptom area, there are three ways to choose an oil:
* One that relates to it on a physical level.
* One that generally helps to balance and heal on a physical or subtle level.
* One that is associated with the nearest energy center.

For example: For a headache, choose an essential oil that is: 1) traditionally used for headaches on a physical level, such as Peppermint; 2) an essential oil that is known to be healing and balancing, such as Lavender; or 3) an essential oil that relates to the Sixth energy center, the Third Eye, such as Basil. Experiment with the different approaches, and use your intuition to decide which approach might be the most useful at any given time. Remember, if you are sincerely drawn to a particular oil for a particular situation, feel free to use it. Then, assess the response.

## AN EXAMPLE OF USING PHYSICAL SYMPTOMS WITH AROMATHERAPY ANOINTING OILS

A man was suffering from muscle pain in his left shoulder. He made a massage oil to warm and ease the discomfort by diluting Rosemary essential oil into a vegetable oil. Every day before he rubbed his shoulder, he put a drop of the massage oil onto his shoulder and visualized a healing, green light radiating out into the shoulder from the point of anointing. He believed that he received greater relief from the massage when it was preceded by an anointing touch.

## CHAPTER FIVE

# AROMATHERAPY ANOINTING FOR CELEBRATIONS & OCCASIONS

*C*reating a ceremony in which to give or receive an aromatherapy anointing is a particularly meaningful way to commemorate special moments in your life—an outward expression of an inner spiritual reality. It can be as simple as lighting a candle and saying an affirmation, or as complex as planning an entire event. The ceremony can be traditional in format, a combination of a variety of traditions, or your own personal creation. It can be designed for just yourself, for one other person, or for a group of people. In all cases, the following steps will help you organize and prepare for the occasion.

## PLANNING YOUR CEREMONY

PLANNING Although some anointing ceremonies are spontaneous, most involve some planning. Identify the theme or purpose of the anointing, make a list of who will attend, and decide where and when it will be. Then determine what special items will be needed, such as candles, incense, or crystals. You may want to review Chapter 3 for ideas.

PREPARATION Make your anointing oil(s). (See Chapter 6.) Gather the special items. Prepare yourself mentally, emotionally, and spiritually.

CLEAN AND ARRANGE Vacuum and dust the area. Clear away any clutter. Arrange chairs or cushions if needed. Place the anointing oil in an area that is easy to access, and place special items where you want them, such as on a table, in the four corners of the room, or surrounding the anointing oil.

CREATE SACRED SPACE As described in Chapter 3, the four steps include clearing the area, protecting the area, asking for guidance, and setting intention. Clear the area before guests arrive. After they are present, protect the area, and then invite guidance to be present. Lastly, declare that the space is for an anointing, and state the intention of the anointing, either silently or aloud.

BODY OF CEREMONY Perform the anointing by putting a drop or two of the anointing oil on the index or middle fingertip of your predominant hand, and then touching the person or object. Every word, action, or component should actualize the full intent of the anointing. The anointing can be accompanied by a blessing, an affirmation, music, dance, or vows. You may also want to invite guests to participate in some way, such as singing or reading together, offering individual blessings, or participating in the actual anointing. For example, at a baptism, everyone could gently anoint the one being baptized.

CLOSE SACRED SPACE

AFTER THE ANOINTING CEREMONY Participants may want to discuss this unique, sacred experience, or simply spend more time together. This is a good time to share a meal. When all is finished, gather your supplies and put things away.

## CELEBRATIONS & OCCASIONS FOR AROMATHERAPY ANOINTING

There are endless opportunities to extend the gift of anointing. Following are eleven general categories of occasions for giving or receiving the blessings of this ancient, sacred technique. They are A Rite of Passage, Place or Object, Healing, Honoring, Love and Devotion, Gratitude, Releasing, Claiming, A Season, A Holiday or Holy Day, and Before an Event.

In each category, there is a list of suggested events and a simple anointing ceremony described for one of those events. The example is intended to help you understand the concept of creating this type of ceremony. It is one that you can try as is, or it may serve to inspire you to create your own. Ceremonies should be personalized so they have true meaning, and we hope that you will embrace this process. For essential oil recommendations per event, see Chapter 6, "Making Aromatherapy Anointing Oils."

## RITE OF PASSAGE

A rite of passage marks a change or an entrance into a new life phase. Examples include a birth, a birthday, death, puberty, becoming a parent, marriage, graduation, a new relationship, divorce, a new job, or becoming an elder (especially at ages 55, 60, or 65). Rite of Passage ceremonies usually include some symbolic action that demonstrates the change or transition such as stepping over a book (symbolic of graduating), or entering into a special circle (symbolic of a new situation such as marriage or becoming an elder).

### RITE OF PASSAGE CEREMONY: BECOMING AN ELDER

FOR A GROUP

* Gather items that represent being an elder to the person who is being celebrated and place them on the floor in a circle formation. These might include books, stones, or pictures of special elders or wonderful old trees. Foods that improve with age, such as cheese or wine, can be included to symbolize the gifts of the aging process.
* Create sacred space. Prepare an aromatherapy anointing oil of Cypress (four drops of the essential oil in one teaspoon of jojoba or olive oil).
* Someone who is already an elder stands inside the circle with the Cypress anointing oil. The celebrated elder stands outside the circle and speaks about what becoming an elder means to them. When ready, she/he steps into the circle. The waiting elder anoints the celebrant with oil on five locations and speaks a blessing, as follows:

ON THE FEET "May you be as sturdy and strong as a healthy, ancient tree."
ON THE HANDS "May all you give and touch convey your wisdom."

ON THE SHOULDERS "May you carry your new responsibilities with ease and grace."

OVER THE HEART "May you be a source of compassionate wisdom, and may your heart be full through all your years."

ON THE SIXTH ENERGY CENTER (BETWEEN THE BROWS) "May the wisdom you have gathered be a source of joy, comfort, and guidance to all who know you."

* The person who is anointing gives a gift to the new elder, anointing the gift with these words: "You are a gift to all people. We welcome and celebrate you."
* The new elder speaks to the participants.
* Each of the participants speaks in appreciation of the new elder.
* Close sacred space, giving thanks. End with clapping and happy sounds. The two elders step together out of the circle and lead the group to a celebration feast.

## PLACE OR OBJECT

Blessing a place, such as a home, office, or piece of land, or blessing an object, such as a piece of cloth, a ring, or a figurine, bestows spiritual significance to an inanimate object. If you are blessing an office or home, anoint each room. If you are blessing a plot of land, anoint the four corners of the property, or draw a symbol in the air while standing in the center of the property. In a ceremony for an object, be certain to anoint the object. If the object is fabric or something that cannot be touched with the anointing oil, anoint your palms, rub them together, and hold them near or around the object.

### PLACE OR OBJECT CEREMONY: A WEDDING RING
FOR A COMMITTED, ENGAGED, OR MARRIED COUPLE

* Create sacred space. Include the ring in this process so that it is cleared of negative energy and protected. Prepare an aromatherapy anointing oil of Elemi (four drops of the essential oil in one teaspoon of jojoba or olive oil).
* Anoint the ring, and state a blessing or affirmation of your intention. For example, "May this ring radiate the love and joy of our marriage," or "This ring is a

reminder of my commitment to my partner." End with a word, such as "Peace" or "Hallelujah."

* Close sacred space, giving thanks.

## HEALING

The definition of the word "healing" is "to make whole in body, mind, and spirit." An aromatherapy anointing for healing may be for yourself, another individual, a group, or an animal. Types of healing include 1) physical, such as a headache; 2) emotional, such as grief; 3) mental, such as confusion; 4) energetic, such as difficulty in communicating; and 5) spiritual, such as feeling disconnected from the Divine.

### HEALING CEREMONY: PHYSICAL
#### FOR YOURSELF OR ONE OTHER PERSON

* Create sacred space. Prepare an aromatherapy anointing oil of Palmarosa (four rops of the essential oil in one teaspoon of jojoba or olive oil).
* Place a drop of Lavender in one of your palms, and rub your hands together to energize them for sending healing energy. Then place the Palmarosa anointing oil on your fingertip and gently anoint the area of the body in need of healing. If it is not possible to touch the area, put the drop of anointing oil on one palm, rub your palms together, and simply hold your hands close to the area—above or around it.
* Rest your hands on or near the area, and imagine healing energy flowing into it.
* Create an image in your mind that represents the physical problem. Then create an image of the problem healing. Bring the two images together and allow the healing image to merge with and overcome the image of the problem.
* Imagine the area now fully healed.
* Sigh as you exhale. Take another breath and say a blessing such as "Thank you for this healing" or an affirmation such as "The healing is now complete."
* Close sacred space, giving thanks.

# HONORING

To honor someone or something is to acknowledge and show respect. Examples of who/what you might honor include elders, ancestors, a marriage, the Earth, the Divine, parents, siblings, children, friends, colleagues, or community members. When honoring a person, include a gift that represents or symbolizes something about that person. For example, if a mother is being honored, give a day at a spa to honor all the giving she has done for others. For a teacher, give a special book to symbolize all the knowledge they have shared. During the ceremony, anoint the gift as well as the person.

## HONORING CEREMONY: EARTH

### WITH YOURSELF, ONE OTHER PERSON, OR A GROUP

* Before creating sacred space, place objects that represent the elements—earth, water, fire, and air—in the four geographical directions of the room. (See Chapter 3 for ideas to represent the elements.) Place the object for air in the east, fire in the south, water in the west, and earth in the north. Then place something in the center that represents the whole earth, such as a living plant, or a globe.

* Create sacred space. Prepare aromatherapy anointing oils of Rosemary, Myrrh, Spikenard, Frankincense, and Vetiver. (Make each one separately: four drops of the essential oil in one teaspoon of jojoba or olive oil.)

* Touch each object with the corresponding anointing oil, saying a blessing or affirmation. Traditionally, begin in the east.

> EAST Anoint with Rosemary. "Bless those who speak the truth about the Earth."
>
> SOUTH Anoint with Myrrh. "Bless those who take care of the Earth."
>
> WEST Anoint with Spikenard. "Bless those who listen to the Earth."
>
> NORTH Anoint with Frankincense. "Bless those who teach the wisdom of the Earth."
>
> CENTER Anoint with Vetiver. "Bless this Earth, which nurtures us. Thank you, dear Mother Earth, for all you provide for us. May you receive all that you need."

* Anoint yourself with Vetiver. "I honor myself as a child of the Earth."
* Close sacred space, giving thanks.

## LOVE AND DEVOTION

The feelings of love and devotion include those of warm-heartedness, personal connection, tenderness, and endearment infused with a sense of commitment. Some examples of those for whom you may feel love and devotion include your companion animals, spouse or life partner, friends, mother, father, siblings, or the Divine.

### LOVE AND DEVOTION CEREMONY: COMPANION ANIMALS
#### FOR YOURSELF AND YOUR ANIMAL FRIEND

* Create sacred space. Prepare an aromatherapy anointing oil of Rose or Tuberose. (four drops of the essential oil in one teaspoon of jojoba or olive oil.)
* Your companion animal should be sitting with you, or held in your lap. If this is not possible, use their picture, or hold an image of them in your mind.
* Speak directly to your animal friend about:
    Why you love them so much.
    How they make you feel.
    Ways in which you show your love to them.
    Your commitment to them.
* Dedicate the relationship with your companion animal to Spirit or the highest good. "May our relationship be for our highest good," or "May the love between us help to foster love everywhere." An affirmation can also be used such as "I devote our companionship to the healing of all animals" or "Our relationship expands my capacity for love and devotion in all realms."
* Anoint yourself on the heart center, and if appropriate or possible, anoint the heart center of your animal friend. Note: If you wish to increase the communication between the two of you, also anoint your Sixth energy center.
* Close sacred space, giving thanks.

## GRATITUDE

Gratitude is an expression of thankfulness and appreciation for someone or something. Examples of who/what you may be grateful for include a job, friends, a home, a spouse or partner, good health, your spiritual community, nourishing food, companion animals, freedom, healing, peace, the resolution of a conflict.

### GRATITUDE CEREMONY: A JOB

FOR YOURSELF

* Create sacred space. Prepare aromatherapy anointing oil of Rose, Bergamot, or Rosemary. (four drops of the essential oil in one teaspoon of jojoba or olive oil.)
* Say a blessing or prayer of thanks. It can be one that you have prepared beforehand, or one that is spontaneous. You may choose to correlate the blessing with one or more energy centers, followed by an anointing, such as:

"I give thanks to Spirit for helping me find this job." (Anoint the Sixth and
        Seventh energy centers.)
"May this job be of benefit to me, my loved ones, and all life." (Anoint the Fourth
        energy center.)
"I dedicate myself to this job with integrity." (Anoint the Third energy center.)
"May my creativity flourish in this job." (Anoint the Second energy center.)
"May this job bring me financial security and abundance." (Anoint the First
        energy center.)

* Close sacred space, giving thanks.

## RELEASING

Releasing refers to the letting go of that which no longer benefits us. Sometimes we are ready to release on all levels—physically, emotionally, mentally, energetically, and spiritually. Other times, we may only be ready to release in stages, on one level or another. Examples of what might be released include the past, illness, outmoded beliefs, lifestyle patterns, emotional wounds, relationships, certain possessions, trauma, or negative emotions such as fear, anger, hatred, or jealousy.

## RELEASING CEREMONY: NEGATIVE EMOTION OF FEAR

### FOR YOURSELF

* Create sacred space. Prepare aromatherapy anointing oils of Juniper and Cedarwood. (Make each separately: four drops of the essential oil in one teaspoon of jojoba or olive oil.)
* Write on a piece of paper the particular negative emotion to be released—in this case, fear.
* Anoint the paper with one drop of the Juniper anointing oil.
* Light the piece of paper with a match or candle, over a fireproof bowl or plate, while saying, "I release my fear," and dropping the paper onto the plate. Allow it to become ash.
* Feel the space you have created within you, free of fear.
* Anoint each of your seven energy centers with Cedarwood and identify what is filling the space created by the release of fear, such as ease, courage, love, joy, or the next phase of your journey. (Whenever we release a negative emotion, we need to fill the emptied space with something positive—an emotion, thought, or image.)
* Close sacred space, giving thanks.

*Note: If it is not possible to use fire, put a drop of Juniper in a bowl of water, and put a pinch of salt into the water as you say your releasing statement. Then pour out the water into a sink or on the ground, with the intention of releasing.*

## CLAIMING

Claiming invites us to fully embody something that we desire, making it a part of who we are. Examples include womanhood, manhood, creativity, power, intuition, sexuality, abundance, health, love, wisdom, faith, or courage. A Claiming Ceremony can be done on its own, or as the second phase of a Releasing Ceremony. Bring an object that represents what you are claiming so that it can be anointed, and then place it in your home or office as a reminder.

### CLAIMING CEREMONY: CREATIVITY

FOR YOURSELF

Choose an object that represents creativity to you. This could be a pen if you are a writer or poet, a paintbrush if you are an artist, or a cookbook if you are a chef.

* Create sacred space. Prepare an aromatherapy anointing oil of Jasmine. (four drops of the essential oil in one teaspoon of jojoba or olive oil.) Place your chosen object in the area.
* Anoint your First, Second, and Fourth energy centers.
* Speak out loud an affirmation or blessing of what you are claiming.

AFFIRMATION EXAMPLES ARE
I claim creativity as my birthright.
I am a creative being.
My creativity is an expression of a joyful heart.
I thoroughly enjoy creative expression.

BLESSING EXAMPLES ARE
May I be a wellspring of creative expression.
Bless my creative nature.
May my creative expression be inspired by Spirit.

* Allow an image or feeling to come to you that represents the creative energy that you are claiming. Anoint your First, Second, and Fourth energy centers again,

imagining that you are placing the image or feeling into your being, completely. Then affirm, "This is true and complete now."

* Close sacred space, giving thanks.

## SEASON

Blessing a particular season shows your appreciation and connects you to the cyclic qualities of nature and life itself. In addition to the seasons, cycles you may choose to celebrate are the solstice, the equinox, or the moon phases.

### SEASON CEREMONY: SPRING

FOR A GROUP

* Create sacred space. Prepare an aromatherapy anointing oil of Geranium. (four drops of the essential oil in one teaspoon of jojoba or olive oil.) Decorate the space with the pastel colors of spring. Participants should wear clothing that represents spring, either by color or style, and bring an object such as a flower that symbolizes spring for them.
* Participants form a circle, and the objects are placed in the center of the circle.
* Choose a person to begin, then go around the circle with each person saying a few words about spring and what it means to them.
* Then go around the circle again with each person anointing the heart center of the person to their right, saying a brief blessing such as, "Bless the new beginnings in your life," or "May you blossom in beauty."
* Say a prayer, sing a song, or read a poem that celebrates and welcomes spring.
* When finished, ring a bell.
* Close sacred space, giving thanks. Share a springtime feast.

## HOLIDAY OR HOLY DAY

A calendar year has many holidays and holy days. An anointing ceremony created specifically to honor the true meaning of Mother's Day, Christmas, Veteran's Day, Hanukkah, or Valentine's Day is a unique way to celebrate it. The area of the ceremony should be decorated with things that represent the holiday or holy day, items that can be anointed as well.

## HOLIDAY CEREMONY: VALENTINE'S DAY

### FOR A COUPLE

Each person brings an object they will give to the other.

* Create sacred space as described in Chapter 3. Each person prepares an anointing oil to exchange. Choose from Rose, Angelica, Bergamot, Jasmine, Lavender, Neroli, Orange, or Rosemary. Review Energy Centers for each of these to help you decide which one to use. (Make each separately: four drops of the essential oil in one teaspoon of jojoba or olive oil.) Sit comfortably across from each other, within easy reach.

* Decide who will begin. The first person anoints the other's heart with the anointing oil, saying, "Let me tell you of my love for you," and continues to express in words their love and affection. When finished, the other person does the same.

* Exchange gifts.

* Anoint each other's gifts with both anointing oils saying, "This gift is a symbol of the love between us."

* Exchange anointing oils.

* Give thanks for the relationship with a blessing, "Thank you for this dear person who is in my life," or an affirmation, "I am grateful for you in my life and for the love between us."

* Give each other a hug or kiss.

* Close sacred space, giving thanks.

## BEFORE AN EVENT

During a day, there is a myriad of events to which anointing can add special significance. Most of them are a part of regular routines such as getting ourselves ready for the day, driving to work, meditating, praying, preparing meals, going to bed, or exercising. There are also special events that occur only once in a while such as interviewing for a new job, having surgery, beginning school, facing a challenging emotional situation, taking an important test, or traveling abroad.

## BEFORE-AN-EVENT CEREMONY: BEGINNING THE DAY
### A PERSONAL STORY

Every morning, Ruah lights a candle to symbolically invite the light of Spirit into her new day. She then walks with piñon incense through her home to clear, cleanse, and bless it. Afterwards, she chooses one of the seven energy-center-anointing blends she has created, to anoint a stone that represents Mother Earth and a crystal that represents Father Sky. She then anoints the center of her body, asking that the oil's teachings infuse her day. Ruah closes her morning ceremony by saying aloud her favorite prayer, "May I be an instrument of your love. May I be an instrument of your will. May I be an instrument of your peace." Finally, she sprays on her favorite essential oil perfume made of Sandalwood, Oakmoss, and Vetiver, and imagines being well-grounded to the Earth, helping her to remain centered and present all day long. She keeps the candle burning until she leaves the house.

## BEFORE-AN-EVENT CEREMONY: VISITING A DYING PERSON
### FOR YOURSELF

* Create sacred space. Prepare an anointing oil. Choose from Azalea, Silver Fir, Mandarin, Myrrh, Orange, Rose, Melissa, or Spikenard. Review the Energy Centers to help you decide which one to use. (four drops of the essential oil in one teaspoon of jojoba or olive oil.)
* Visualize the person you will be visiting. Allow yourself to experience all your feelings, especially the difficult ones.
* Gently anoint your Second energy center, visualizing all the emotions that connect you with the person you will be visiting. Honor the relationship, and ask that anything needing to be healed between the two of you be healed.

* With a breath, blow any negativity into the earth or up to the sun.

* Anoint your heart, speaking an affirmation that blesses the person and your relationship with them. For example, "I bring love and support to you for your journey," or "May there be peace and gentle release between us," or "I honor your journey and I let you go with love," or "May your transition be peaceful and filled with light."

* Anoint your hands, rub them together, and move your arms around your body to create a grounded, compassionate circle of protected emotional authenticity, mental clarity, and compassionate presence. Bless or affirm yourself as a source of support for this person and any others present: "I will do my best to support this process," or "Help me to be a support during this time of need."

* Close sacred space, giving thanks.

## CHAPTER SIX
# MAKING AROMATHERAPY
# ANOINTING OILS

*M*aking aromatherapy anointing oils is easy, fun, and rewarding. The process adds a further dimension to the meaningfulness of anointing, no matter what the occasion. It also allows you, through personal experience, to learn about and enjoy the captivating world of essential oils.

The standard proportion for making an anointing oil is four drops of essential oil to one teaspoon of vegetable oil. If you would prefer to minimize the fragrance of an essential oil (not all of them may be to your liking), or if you are using a strong oil that may irritate the skin such as Cinnamon, use only one or two drops to a teaspoon of vegetable oil. If you prefer to have the fragrance more apparent and are using a gentle oil such as Lavender or Rose, try ten drops to a teaspoon. On an energetic level, any of these formulas will work well. If you are not familiar with the strength of essential oils on the skin, you should invest in one of the aromatherapy books listed in Resources as a guide.

To make aromatherapy anointing oils, you will need the following supplies:

* A measuring spoon—teaspoon size.
* The chosen essential oil for the particular purpose of the anointing. We recommend having a selection of essential oils on hand. A good, basic collection includes Lavender, Rose, Sandalwood, Cedarwood, Vetiver, Orange, German Chamomile, Juniper, Clary Sage, and Jasmine.
* A vegetable oil, such as jojoba, olive, or sesame.

\* A small glass bottle with a tight-fitting cap. (Dark-colored glass—amber or cobalt blue—is preferred to protect the oil from ultraviolet light.)

Once you have collected your supplies, follow these three simple steps:

\* Create sacred space as described in Chapter 3—clear the area, protect the area, ask for guidance, and set intention. Pay particular attention to your intention, naming the purpose of the anointing oil.

\* Put the essential oils in the little bottle. Add the vegetable oil. Put the cap on and gently shake the bottle or roll it in your hands. As you are holding it, imbue it with positive thoughts and good feelings.

\* Bless the finished oil: "May this anointing oil always be in service to the highest good," or "Bless this oil so that it may _____ *(fill in your intention)."*

Though the steps to make an anointing oil are simple, each one is important and contributes to the quality of the finished product. Make anointing oils when you have ample time and are not in a hurry, and only when you are in a positive state of mind.

## VEGETABLE OILS

Vegetable oils have a rich, emollient quality that is ideal for blending with essential oils. When used to dilute essential oils, they are commonly called carrier or base oils. Though there are many more carrier oils than the ones listed below, these are the preferred ones for anointing, with jojoba and olive being the top choices.

\* Jojoba oil is actually more of a liquid wax than it is an oil. Because of this, its rich texture resists rancidity, staying fresh for long periods of time. Energetically, it draws the essential oils into the body to be distributed.

\* Olive oil is a rich, fragrant oil that has been traditionally used for anointing. Energetically, it affects all levels simultaneously—the physical, emotional, mental, and spiritual.

\* Sesame oil is a medium-weight oil that has been used since ancient times. Energetically, it helps to align all the energy centers.

* Canola oil is a medium-weight oil that is popular for massage. Energetically, it has an illuminating quality—bringing light into darkness.
* Hazelnut oil is a finely textured, lightweight oil that is quickly absorbed by the skin. Energetically, it is grounding and supports the working together of spirit and body.
* Sunflower oil is a medium-weight oil that has been treasured since ancient times. Energetically, it is particularly good for assisting with emotional healing.

## ESSENTIAL OILS FOR AROMATHERAPY ANOINTING OCCASIONS

Following are the eleven categories of occasions for creating anointing oils, as discussed in Chapter 5. There is a list of examples for each of the eleven categories of anointing occasions, followed by suggested single essential oils. The suggestions are not all-inclusive—there are other oils that will work well for each example. This list is intended to provide you with a place to begin. Read about the suggested oils in Chapter 2 to help you choose the best oil for your situation. As always, we encourage you to explore, experiment, and discover the essential oils that work for you.

### ESSENTIAL OILS FOR RITES OF PASSAGE
GENERAL (USEFUL FOR ALL OCCASIONS INVOLVING CHANGE) Cypress
BIRTH Frangipani, Lavender
BIRTHDAY Frankincense, Ginger, Vetiver
DEATH Melissa, Bergamot, Ylang Ylang
PUBERTY Roman Chamomile, Fennel, Ylang Ylang
BECOMING A PARENT Calamus, Mandarin, Vetiver
MARRIAGE German Chamomile, Jasmine, Rose
GRADUATION Roman Chamomile, Erigeron
BECOMING AN ELDER Benzoin, Cedarwood, Cypress
BEGINNING A NEW RELATIONSHIP Silver Fir, Rose, Rosemary
DIVORCE Cypress, Lemon, Myrrh, Rose
NEW JOB Guaiac Wood, Oakmoss

## ESSENTIAL OILS FOR PLACES AND OBJECTS

GENERAL (USEFUL FOR ALL PLACES AND THINGS) Vetiver, Oakmoss

A HOME Angelica, Rose, Vetiver

A PLACE OF WORK Calamus, Sea Fennel

A PIECE OF LAND Frangipani, Hay, Leptospermum, Oakmoss

A TREASURED OBJECT Cedarwood, Frangipani, Ginger, Elemi

## ESSENTIAL OILS FOR HEALING

GENERAL (USEFUL FOR ALL SITUATIONS INVOLVING HEALING)
Lavender, Palmarosa, Vetiver

PHYSICAL Coriander, Frangipani, Mastic, Vetiver, Palmarosa

EMOTIONAL Azalea, Bergamot, Eucalyptus, Silver Fir, Mandarin, Myrrh, Rose,
Ylang Ylang

MENTAL Anise, Bay Laurel, Copaiva Balm, Lemon, Neroli

ENERGETIC Champaca, Fennel, Juniper, Sea Fennel

SPIRITUAL Calamus, Cedarwood, Cypress, Erigeron, Frankincense,
Rosewood, Sandalwood

## ESSENTIAL OILS FOR HONORING

GENERAL (USEFUL FOR ALL OCCASIONS INVOLVING HONORING)
Frankincense, Rosemary

ELDERS Guaiac Wood, Vetiver

ANCESTORS Rosemary, Leptospermum

MARRIAGE German Chamomile, Jasmine, Sandalwood

EARTH Cedarwood, Vetiver, Patchouli, Rosemary, Myrrh, Spikenard, Frankincense

THE DIVINE Angelica, Lavender

PARENTS Frankincense, Rose

SIBLINGS Orange, Rose, Jasmine

CHILDREN Orange, Cajeput

COLLEAGUES Fennel

FRIEND Rose, Tuberose

## ESSENTIAL OILS FOR LOVE AND DEVOTION

GENERAL (USEFUL FOR ALL OCCASIONS INVOLVING LOVE) Rose,
Spikenard, Tuberose

COMPANION ANIMALS Benzoin, Orange, Lavender, Cajeput, Vetiver,
Rose, Tuberose

SPOUSE OR PARTNER Bergamot, Rose, Ylang Ylang, German and
Roman Chamomile, Fennel, Jasmine

FRIENDS Lavender, Bergamot, Mandarin, Orange

MOTHER Frangipani, Jasmine, Rose, Myrrh

FATHER Ginger, Rosemary, Sandalwood, Myrrh

SIBLINGS Rose, Ginger, Orange

THE DIVINE Rosemary, Sandalwood, Cedarwood, Frankincense, Vetiver

## ESSENTIAL OILS FOR GRATITUDE

GENERAL (USEFUL FOR ALL OCCASIONS INVOLVING GRATITUDE)
Ginger, Angelica, Cajeput, Rose, Frankincense, Orange, Jasmine, Lavender,
Bergamot, Mandarin, Sandalwood, Vetiver, Rosemary

## ESSENTIAL OILS FOR RELEASING

GENERAL (USEFUL FOR ALL OCCASIONS INVOLVING RELEASING)
Juniper, Cedarwood

PAST Lavender, Cypress, Neroli, Vetiver

ILLNESS Coriander, Palmarosa

OUTMODED BELIEFS Anise, Bay Laurel, Juniper, Lemon, Elemi

LIFESTYLE PATTERNS Copaiva Balm, Guaiac Wood, Mandarin

EMOTIONAL WOUNDS Azalea, Silver Fir, Myrrh, Spikenard, Bergamot

RELATIONSHIPS Jasmine, Juniper, Melissa, Rose, Frankincense

CERTAIN POSSESSIONS Cedarwood, Ginger, Cypress, Rosemary

TRAUMA Benzoin, Cypress, Frankincense, Spikenard, Lavender, Ylang Ylang

NEGATIVE EMOTIONS

GENERAL (USEFUL FOR ALL SITUATIONS INVOLVING NEGATIVE EMOTIONS)
Azalea, Eucalyptus, Vetiver

FEAR Azalea, Fennel, Spikenard, Ylang Ylang, Juniper, Cedarwood

ANGER Ylang Ylang, Bergamot, Rose

HATRED Eucalyptus, Rose

JEALOUSY Cypress, Ylang Ylang

## ESSENTIAL OILS FOR CLAIMING

GENERAL (USEFUL FOR ALL TYPES OF CLAIMING) Sandalwood,
Rosewood, Oakmoss

WOMANHOOD Jasmine, Frangipani

MANHOOD Jasmine, Ginger, Bay Laurel

CREATIVITY Clary Sage, Orange, Jasmine

POWER Black Pepper, Fennel, Neroli, Sea Fennel, Ylang Ylang

INTUITION Immortelle, Lemon, Clary Sage, Rosewood, Elemi

SEXUALITY Ginger, Jasmine, Sandalwood, Rose

ABUNDANCE Ginger, Oakmoss, Vetiver

HEALTH Coriander, Mastic, Palmarosa

LOVE Jasmine, Rose, Spikenard, Elemi

WISDOM Calamus, Cedarwood, German Chamomile, Leptospermum, Monarda,
Rosemary, Frankincense

FAITH Angelica, Sandalwood, Cajeput

COURAGE Ginger, Juniper, Myrrh

## ESSENTIAL OILS FOR A SEASON

GENERAL (USEFUL FOR ALL OCCASIONS INVOLVING A SEASON) Leptospermum

SPRING Erigeron, Hay, Geranium

SUMMER Orange, Oakmoss

FALL Cypress, Ginger

WINTER Frankincense, Vetiver

SOLSTICE Cedarwood, Jasmine

EQUINOX Frangipani, Lavender

MOON CYCLES

   NEW MOON Clary Sage, Anise

   FULL MOON Guaiac Wood, Ginger

## ESSENTIAL OILS FOR A HOLIDAY OR HOLY DAY

GENERAL (USEFUL FOR ALL OCCASIONS INVOLVING A HOLIDAY OR HOLY DAY)
   Orange, Cedarwood

MOTHER'S DAY Rose, Frangipani, Jasmine

FATHER'S DAY Ginger, Rose, Sandalwood

PASSOVER Cypress, Juniper, Melissa

CHRISTMAS Frankincense, Myrrh

EASTER Angelica, Cedarwood, Guaiac Wood, Melissa

VETERAN'S DAY German Chamomile, Myrrh

VALENTINE'S DAY Rose, Angelica, Bergamot, Jasmine, Lavender, Neroli,
   Orange, Rosemary

SABBATH Rose, Angelica, Benzoin, Sandalwood, Gurjum

MEMORIAL DAY Melissa, Anise, Lavender, Myrrh

RAMADAN Frankincense, Cedarwood, Myrrh

THANKSGIVING Ginger, Geranium, Neroli

HANUKKAH Angelica, Cedarwood

ESSENTIAL OILS FOR BEFORE AN EVENT

GENERAL (USEFUL BEFORE ANY EVENT) Vetiver, Sandalwood, Lavender

DAILY COMMUTE Cypress, Azalea, Mastic

BEGINNING THE DAY Champaca, Lavender, Vetiver, Sandalwood

MEDITATION / PRAYER Cedarwood, Frankincense, Lavender, Champaca, Gurjum

PREPARING MEALS Frangipani, Geranium

GOING TO SLEEP AT NIGHT Clary Sage, Cedarwood

PHYSICAL ACTIVITY Vetiver, Orange, Mastic, Palmarosa

JOB INTERVIEW Lemon, German Chamomile, Erigeron, Oakmoss

GETTING MARRIED Rose, Jasmine, Sandalwood, Orange

SURGERY Coriander, Lavender, Palmarosa

BEGINNING SCHOOL Rosemary, Lemon, Copaiva Balm

EMOTIONAL SITUATION Azalea, Silver Fir, Mandarin, Myrrh, Orange,
Rose, Spikenard

MENTAL CHALLENGE Rosemary, Lemon, Copaiva Balm, Fennel,
Immortelle, Neroli

TRAVELING ABROAD Cypress, German Chamomile, Anise

## CREATING BLENDS FOR AROMATHERAPY ANOINTING OILS

Instead of using a single essential oil for your anointing oil, you may choose to use a blend of essential oils. Use as many as you like, but stay within the formulation guide-lines—one to ten drops of essential oil per teaspoon of vegetable oil, depending on the oils used and your preference for strength of fragrance. Following are a few blends for you to try, and we encourage you to create your own.

AROMATHERAPY ANOINTING OIL FOR STARTING A NEW JOB

2 drops Cypress for change and confidence

1 drop Guaiac Wood for finding one's life work and purpose

1 drop Oakmoss for an increased sense of prosperity

1 teaspoon jojoba or olive oil

## AROMATHERAPY ANOINTING OIL FOR YOUR HOME

1 drop Angelica to encourage the presence of angels

2 drops Rose to create the intention of a loving home

1 drop Vetiver to protect the home from negative influences

1 teaspoon jojoba or olive oil

## AROMATHERAPY ANOINTING OIL FOR EMOTIONAL HEALING

3 drops Bergamot for optimism

1 drop Rose to support the heart center and promote love, hope, and patience

1 teaspoon jojoba or olive oil

## AROMATHERAPY ANOINTING OIL FOR HONORING A MARRIAGE

1 drop German Chamomile to support calm, truthful communication

2 drops Jasmine to promote love and sensuality, and to unite the masculine and feminine

1 drop Sandalwood to ground and to open the heart to trust and love

1 teaspoon jojoba or olive oil

## AROMATHERAPY ANOINTING OIL FOR LOVE AND DEVOTION TO ONE'S MOTHER

1 drop Frangipani to heal the relationship with your mother

1 drop Rose to express love and compassion

1 drop Jasmine to warm and open the heart

1 drop Myrrh to strengthen the relationship with your mother

1 teaspoon jojoba or olive oil

## AROMATHERAPY ANOINTING OIL FOR GRATITUDE TOWARDS YOUR COMPANION ANIMAL

1 drop Rose for unconditional love

3 drops Orange for joy

1 teaspoon jojoba or olive oil

### AROMATHERAPY ANOINTING OIL FOR RELEASING A RELATIONSHIP

2 drops Rose for healing wounds of the heart

1 drop Frankincense to stabilize the emotions

1 drop Melissa to promote emotional clarity

1 teaspoon jojoba or olive oil

### AROMATHERAPY ANOINTING OIL FOR CLAIMING CREATIVITY

1 drop Clary Sage for inspiration

2 drops Orange for self-confidence and joy

1 drop Jasmine to enhance intuition

1 teaspoon jojoba or olive oil

### AROMATHERAPY ANOINTING OIL FOR THE WINTER SEASON

2 drops Vetiver to acknowledge the wisdom of winter

2 drops Frankincense to acknowledge this time of rest and "going inward"

1 teaspoon jojoba or olive oil

### AROMATHERAPY ANOINTING OIL FOR FATHER'S DAY

2 drops Rose for healing emotional wounds and expressing unconditional love

2 drops Sandalwood to acknowledge the sense of security a father offers

1 teaspoon jojoba or olive oil

### AROMATHERAPY ANOINTING OIL FOR MEDITATION

2 drops Cedarwood to calm and steady the mind

1 drop Frankincense to ground, center, and deepen the breath

1 drop Champaca to balance all the energy centers

1 teaspoon jojoba or olive oil

# RESOURCES

## CHAPTER ONE

### JUDY ZOLEZZI
Judy is a massage therapist and spiritual director. She teaches classes on "Massage as Anointing—Honoring the Body as Sacred" and offers retreats and workshops on personal/spiritual growth for women and men. 831-475-3969

### BARBRA TELYNOR
Barbra is a singer, harpist, contemporary ceremonialist, and teacher. She is an ordained minister in the United Church of Christ. She is available for guidance and for weddings and other personal and community ceremony experiences. 831-465-9698

### LAURA BINAH FELDMAN
Laura Binah Feldman is available to create and facilitate multicultural, interfaith rituals for life-cycle and seasonal celebrations. Pomegranate House, 831-479-7578

### PHYLLIS WILLIAMS
Phyllis is an intuitive nutritionist, health awareness specialist, and Reiki practitioner. She is the author of *How to Choose the Perfect Color for Your Candles* and *Candle Rituals for the New Millennium*. She teaches candle ritual classes and workshops. 707-967-0620

### JAN BODDIE AND MARYSTELLA CHURCH
Jan offers spiritual healing and celebrations through rituals, retreats, personalized rites of passage, classes, and consultation. Marystella is in private practice as an intuitive

energy healer and works with groups as a ritualist and educator. New Moons Sacred Sight Journeys, 707-542-4928

THE REVEREND MARGO BEARHEART
Margo is the founder and director of the Transformational and Healing Arts Center in Santa Rosa, California. She teaches classes in energy healing, medical intuition, shamanic studies, and personal spiritual growth. 707-579-0737

## CHAPTER TWO

### AROMATHERAPY EDUCATION

LIGHT-TOUCHED™
Ruah Bull and Joni Keim Loughran
PO BOX 750986
Petaluma, CA 94975
707-573-6071 or 707-765-6986
www.light-touched.com

TWIN LAKES COLLEGE OF THE HEALING ARTS
Aromatherapy Program
1210 Brommer Street
Santa Cruz, CA 95062
831-476-2152

COLLEGE OF BOTANICAL HEALING ARTS
Elizabeth Van Buren
1821 Seventh Avenue
Santa Cruz, CA 95062
831-462-1807

MICHAEL SCHOLES SCHOOL OF AROMATIC STUDIES
4218 N. Glencoe, No. 4
Marina Del Rey, CA 90292
310-827-7737

Contact the National Association of Holistic Aromatherapy (NAHA) at
888-ASK-NAHA for a list of national and international aromatherapy schools.

ESSENTIAL OILS

Many excellent aromatherapy companies offer therapeutic-quality essential oils. We
use oils from a variety of sources and particularly recommend those that have not been
exposed to electromagnetic machinery, which can disrupt the subtle properties. This
is especially important when using essential oils for their vibrational qualities. The following companies take these protective measures.

OSHADHI USA
1340-G Industrial Avenue
Petaluma, CA 94952
707-763-0662

FRAGRANT EARTH
2000 Second Avenue, No. 206
Seattle, WA 98121
206-374-8773

BOOKS ON AROMATHERAPY

*Aromatherapy & Subtle Energy Techniques,* Joni Keim Loughran and Ruah Bull
    (Berkeley, CA: Frog, Ltd., 2000).
*Aromatherapy for Healing the Spirit,* Gabriel Mojay (New York: Henry Holt and
    Company, 1996).

*Fragrant Mind,* Valerie Ann Worwood (Novato, CA: New World Publishing, 1999.)

*Subtle Aromatherapy,* Patricia Davis (England: C. W. Daniel Company Limited, 1991).

*Aromatherapy for Vibrant Health and Beauty,* Roberta Wilson (Garden City Park, NY: Avery Publishing Group, 1995).

*The Illustrated Encyclopedia of Essential Oils,* Julia Lawless (Rockport, MA: Element Books, 1995).

## AROMATHERAPY ASSOCIATIONS

### NATIONAL ASSOCIATION OF HOLISTIC AROMATHERAPY

1-888-ASK-NAHA

## BOOKS ON AFFIRMATIONS

*Affirmations,* Cathy Guiswite (New York: Andrews and McMeel, 1996).

*Affirmations,* Stuart Wilde, Jill Kramer (Carlsbad, CA: Hay House, Inc., 1993).

## CHAPTER THREE

### BOOKS ON AROMATHERAPY

See Resources for Chapter 2.

### BOOKS ON BLESSINGS / PRAYERS

*Healing Words,* Larry Dossey (New York: HarperCollins, 1993).

*Prayers for Healing,* ed. Maggie Oman (Berkeley, CA: Conari Press, 1997).

*Earth Prayers,* ed. Elizabeth Roberts and Elias Amidor (San Francisco: Harper, 1991).

*Life Prayers,* ed. Elizabeth Roberts and Elias Amidor (San Francisco: Harper, 1996).

## BOOKS ON CANDLES
*Candle Power,* Phyllis Williams and Dorothy Breitenstein (Calistoga, CA: Candle
  Power Company, 1999). PO BOX 164, Calistoga, CA 94515
*Candles, Meditations, and Healing,* Charlene Whitaker (New York: Llewellyn
  Publishing, 2000).

## BOOKS ON COLORS
*The Healing Power of Color,* Betty Wood (Rochester, VT: Destiny Books, 1992).
*Color Your Life,* Howard and Dorothy Sun (New York: Ballantine Books, 1992).
*Color and Crystals: A Journey Through the Chakras,* Joy Gardner-Gordon (Freedom,
  CA: Crossing Press, 1988).

## BOOKS ON CRYSTALS / STONES
*Healing with Gemstones and Crystals,* Diane Stein (Freedom, CA: Crossing Press, 1996).
*Crystal Enlightenment,* Katrina Raphaell (New York: Aurora Press, 1985).
*The Complete Crystal Guidebook,* Uma Sibley (San Francisco: U-Read Publications, 1986).
*Color and Crystals: A Journey Through the Chakras,* Joy Gardner-Gordon (Freedom,
  CA: Crossing Press, 1988).

## BOOKS ON THE ELEMENTS
*Four-Fold Way,* Angeles Arrien (San Francisco: Harper, 1993).
*Earth Medicine,* Kenneth Meadows (Rockport, MA: Element Books, 1989).

## BOOKS ON FLOWER ESSENCES
*Flowers That Heal,* Patricia Kaminski (Dublin: New Leaf, 1998). Available from
  Flower Essence Society, Nevada City, CA  Phone: 530-265-9163.

*Flower Remedies Handbook,* Donna Cunningham (New York: Sterling Publishing Co., Inc., 1992).

*Flower Power,* Anne McIntyre (New York: Henry Holt and Company, 1996).

BOOKS ON SACRED SPACE

*Sacred Space,* Denise Linn (New York: Ballantine Books, 1995).

*Creating Sacred Space with Feng Shui,* Karen Kingston and Denise Linn (New York: Broadway Publishing, 1997).

BOOKS ON SOUNDS

*The Book of Sound Therapy,* Olivea Dewhurst-Maddock (New York: Simon and Schuster, 1993).

*Healing Mantra, Using Sound Affirmations for Personal Power,* Thomas Ashley-Farrand (New York: Ballantine, 1999).

*Sounds of Healing,* Mitchell L. Gaynor (New York: Broadway Books, 1999).

BOOKS ON VIBRATIONAL HEALING

*Vibrational Medicine for the 21st Century,* Richard Gerber, MD. (New York: HarperCollins, 2000).

BOOKS ON VISUALIZATIONS

*Creative Visualization,* Shakti Gawain (Berkeley, CA: Whatever Publishing, 1978).

*Secrets of Creative Visualization,* Phillip Cooper (New York: Samuel Weiser, Inc., 1999).

*Rituals of Healing: Using Imagery for Health & Wellness,* Jeanne Achterberg, Barbara Dossey, Leslie Kolkmeier (New York: Bantam Books, 1994).

# CHAPTER FOUR

## BOOKS ON BODY SYMBOLOGY
*You Can Heal Your Life,* Louise L. Hay (Carlsbad, CA: Hay House, Inc., 1987).
*The Healing Power of Illness,* Thorwald Dethlefsen and Rütiger Dahlke (Rockport, MA: Element Books, 1990).

## BOOKS ON SUBTLE ANATOMY
*Wheels of Life,* Anodea Judith (St. Paul, MN: Llewellyn Publishing, 1996).
*Wheels of Light,* Rosalyn Bruyere (New York: Fireside Books, 1994).
*Hands of Light,* Barbara Brennan (New York: Bantam Books, 1988).

## BOOKS ON TOUCH
*Touching: The Human Significance of Skin,* Ashley Montagu (New York: Harper & Row, 1986).
*A Gift for Healing,* Deborah Cowens (New York: Crown Trade Paperbacks, 1996).
*Hands on Healing,* Jack Angelo (Rochester, VT: Healing Arts Press, 1997).
*Your Hands Can Heal,* Ric A. Weinman (New York: Penguin Books, 1992).

# CHAPTER FIVE

## BOOKS ON CEREMONIES
*Ritual: Power of Healing & the Spirit,* Malidoma Somé (New York: Penguin Books, 1997).
*The Power of Ritual,* Rachel Pollack (New York: Dell Publishing, 2000).

*Circle Left to Enter Rite,* Jan Boddie, PHD. (Santa Rosa, CA: New Moon Sacred Sight Journeys Publishing, 1996).

## CHAPTER SIX

### SOURCES FOR ESSENTIAL OILS
See Resources for Chapter 2

### SOURCES FOR GLASS BOTTLES
SKS
Bottle and Packaging, Inc.
518-899-7488

### SOURCES FOR ORGANIC CARRIER OILS
NATURAL FOOD STORES

OSHADHI USA
707-763-0662

# SAFETY GUIDELINES FOR USING ESSENTIALS OILS

* Do not take essential oils internally.
* Keep essential oils tightly closed and away from children.
* Keep essential oils away from and out of your eyes. (If this should occur, first put a drop of carrier oil such as canola or sweet almond in your eye to collect the essential oil. If no carrier oil is available, rinse extremely well with water.)
* Dilute essential oils before applying them to the skin.
* Citrus oils can cause sensitivity and discoloration of the skin when exposed to direct sunlight.
* If you are allergy-prone, test the oil under a bandage for 12 hours. If there is no reaction, the oil should be safe to use. If there is swelling or irritation, do not use the oil.
* If your skin becomes irritated with essential oils, rub the area with a vegetable oil and discontinue use.
* If you are pregnant, there are many oils you should not use. Use a reference book.
* If you have a heart condition, there are oils you should not use. Use a reference book.
* If you are taking homeopathic remedies, essential oils may negate their effect. Check with your physician.
* If you have epilepsy, do not use essential oils without consulting your physician.
* If you have asthma, do not inhale essential oils without medical direction.
* Don't put essential oils near a flame—they are flammable.

# GLOSSARY OF TERMS

## BALANCED
A healthy state. When all aspects—physical, psychological, and spiritual—work together harmoniously. Unbalanced: when one or more aspects are not in a healthy state, causing disharmony as a whole.

## BEING PRESENT
Awareness of the here and now, grounded and centered.

## BLOCKS (PHYSICAL, MENTAL, EMOTIONAL, ENERGETIC)
When thoughts, emotions, and/or physical sensations are unable to manifest or be experienced, causing a state of stagnation in the flow of energy. More specifically referred to as physical blocks, mental blocks, emotional blocks, and energy blocks.

## BOUNDARIES
The encompassing of our psychological and energetic being. Defines what we do and do not want, or will and will not allow, in our lives. For example, "It is unacceptable for you to speak to me in that tone of voice." Boundary statements are often followed by consequences, "If you continue to speak to me that way I will ask you to leave." Healthy boundaries allow influence from that which nurtures and supports us and keeps out that which does not.

## CENTERED
The body/mind experience of being in the body, in the present moment, alert, aware, and responsive. Being centered often has a kinesthetic quality that could be described as "I am me, fully here, fully awake."

### ENERGY
Subtle energy medicine teaches that all life forms radiate and are composed of energy. This energy, also referred to as life force, creates and maintains our life and physical being, similar to the charge in a battery. When this energy is depleted, blocked, or distorted in some way, it can result in imbalance, illness, or death.

### GROUNDED
A sense of stability and solidity. Something that connects us energetically to Earth to create a sense of conscious awareness and physical presence.

### GUIDANCE
Direction, help, assistance, advice, counsel. Spiritual guidance can be from someone or something on the physical plane, such as a person, plant, or book, or on the non-physical plane, such as Buddha, Christ, angels, or someone who has died. It is experienced in a variety of ways such as a physical sensation, a vision, an inner voice, an outer voice, or an impression in the heart center or mind. Highest guidance is received directly from the Divine.

### HEAL
Derived from the Anglo-Saxon word "haelen" which means "to make whole." To be in balance in mind, body, and spirit.

### HEALING ENERGY
Life force energy generated in the spiritual realm that supports healing on any level—physical, mental, emotional, or spiritual.

### HIGHER SELF
The part of a person that is evolved and connected to the Divine.

### INNER CHILD
That aspect of the psyche that carries and remembers the experiences, wounds, and gifts of who we were as children.

PATH

"The path" is a metaphor for our religious or spiritual journey through life. It includes everything that involves our spirituality, such as our beliefs, practices, and experiences. It is often referred to as "chosen path" or "spiritual path."

SPIRITUAL

That which is about the larger, mysterious, transpersonal realm. It may or may not have a religious format. Spirituality: An awareness of that larger realm, beyond the personal.

RELEASE

To let go of blocks so that energy can flow, whether they be physical, mental, emotional, or energetic.

RELIGION

A faith tradition that includes beliefs (theology), practices (ritual, both personal and communal), and a connection to a historical and present-day community.

THOUGHTFORMS

Energy bundles created by thoughts, especially habitual thoughts. Metaphysically, thoughts that become an actual energetic object, capable of impact on any level—physical, emotional, mental, and spiritual. They usually represent our perceptions and beliefs about reality, determine how we experience life, and draw experiences to us that confirm our belief system.

# INDEX

Beliefs, outmoded, 17, 20, 54–55, 133
Benzoin (Styrax benzoe), 21–22
Bergamot (Citrus bergamia), 22–24
Biofield, 13–14
Birth, 131
Birthday, 131
Black Pepper (Piper nigrum), 24–25
Blessings, 15, 90–91, 142. See also
    individual oils
Boddie, Jan, 7–8, 94, 139–40
Body
    accepting, 23
    strengthening, 61
Body symbology, 105–7, 145
Boswellia carterii. See Frankincense
Breath, 44–45
Brennan, Barbara, 14
Brow Center, 110
Bruyere, Rosalyn, 57
Buddha, 3, 88, 97
Buddhism, 13, 16, 75
Bulnesia sarmienti. See Guaiac Wood
Burn-out, 40, 61

C
Cajeput (Melaleuca cajuputii), 25–26
Calamus (Acorus calamus), 26–27
Cananga odorata. See Ylang Ylang
Canarium luzonicum. See Elemi
Candles, 91, 143
Canola oil, 131
Carrier oils, 146

Cedarwood (Cedrus atlantica), 8, 27–28, 87
Ceremonies, 115–28
    books on, 145–46
    claiming, 124–25, 134
    before an event, 126–28, 136
    gratitude, 122, 133
    healing, 119, 132
    holiday or holy day, 125–26, 135
    honoring, 120–21, 132–33
    love and devotion, 121, 133
    place or object, 118–19, 132
    planning, 115–16
    releasing, 122–23, 133–34
    rite of passage, 117–18, 131
    season, 125, 135
Chakras. See Energy centers
Chamomile, German (Chamomilla
    matricaria), 29–30
Chamomile, Roman (Anthemis
    nobilis), 30–31
Champaca (Michelia champaca), 31–32
Change, 25, 36, 39, 85
Cherokee, 94
Childhood issues, 60
Children, honoring, 132
Chinese medicine, 94
Christianity, 1–2, 13, 16, 98
Christmas, 135
Church, Marystella, 7–8, 94, 139–40
Citrus aurantium. See Neroli; Orange
Citrus bergamia. See Bergamot
Citrus limonum. See Lemon